Julianna Abrams

Diabetic Diet After 50

for Beginners

Healthy Diabetics Diet Recommendations with nutritional guidelines, Delicious Low-Sugar & Low-Carb Suggestions and Full Color Pictures

"Dedicated to my dad and to everyone like him who must face with and manage this little monster, with strength, determination, and courage."

⭐ BONUS ⭐

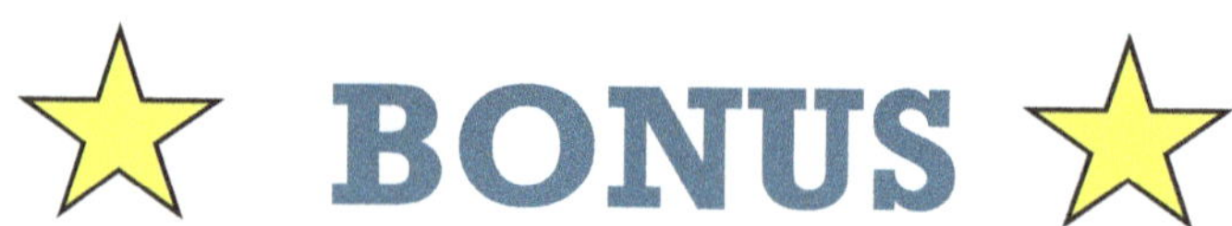

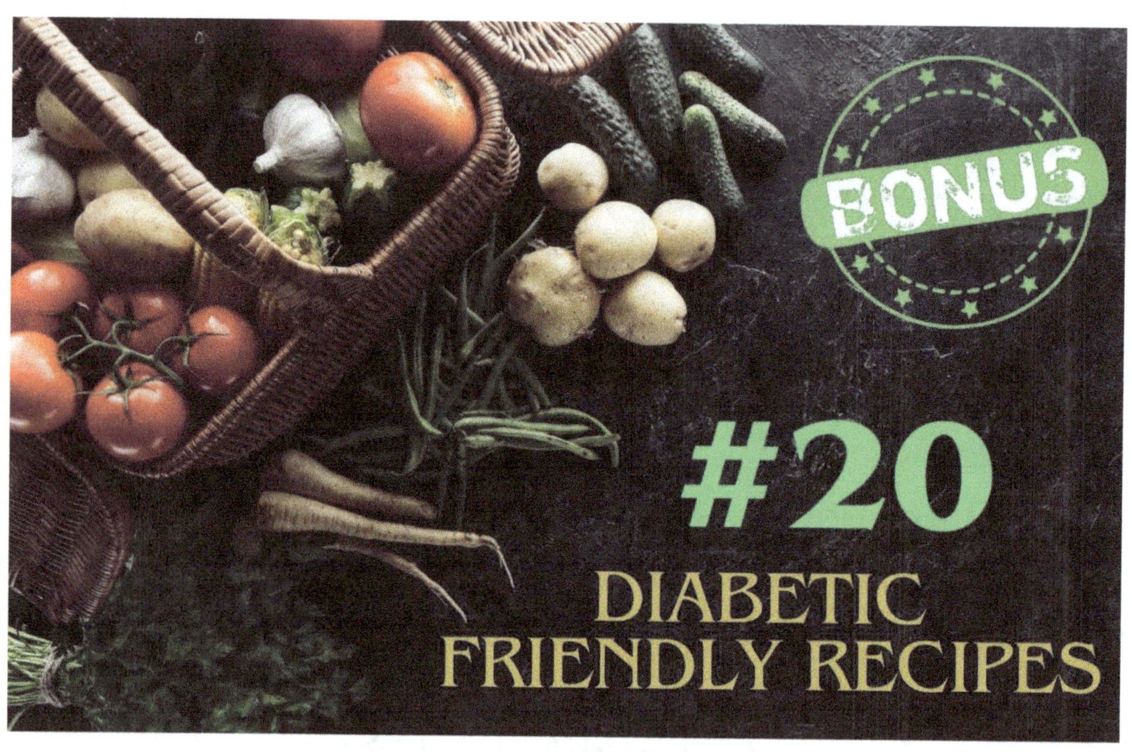

SCROLL TO THE END AND

SCAN THE QR CODE

TABLE OF CONTENTS:

CHAPTER 17: 104

MEAL PREP FOR SPECIAL OCCASIONS 104

CHAPTER 18: 109

STAYING MOTIVATED ON YOUR MEAL PREP JOURNEY 109

CHAPTER 19: 115

RESOURCES FOR CONTINUED LEARNING 115

CONCLUSION 121

Introduction

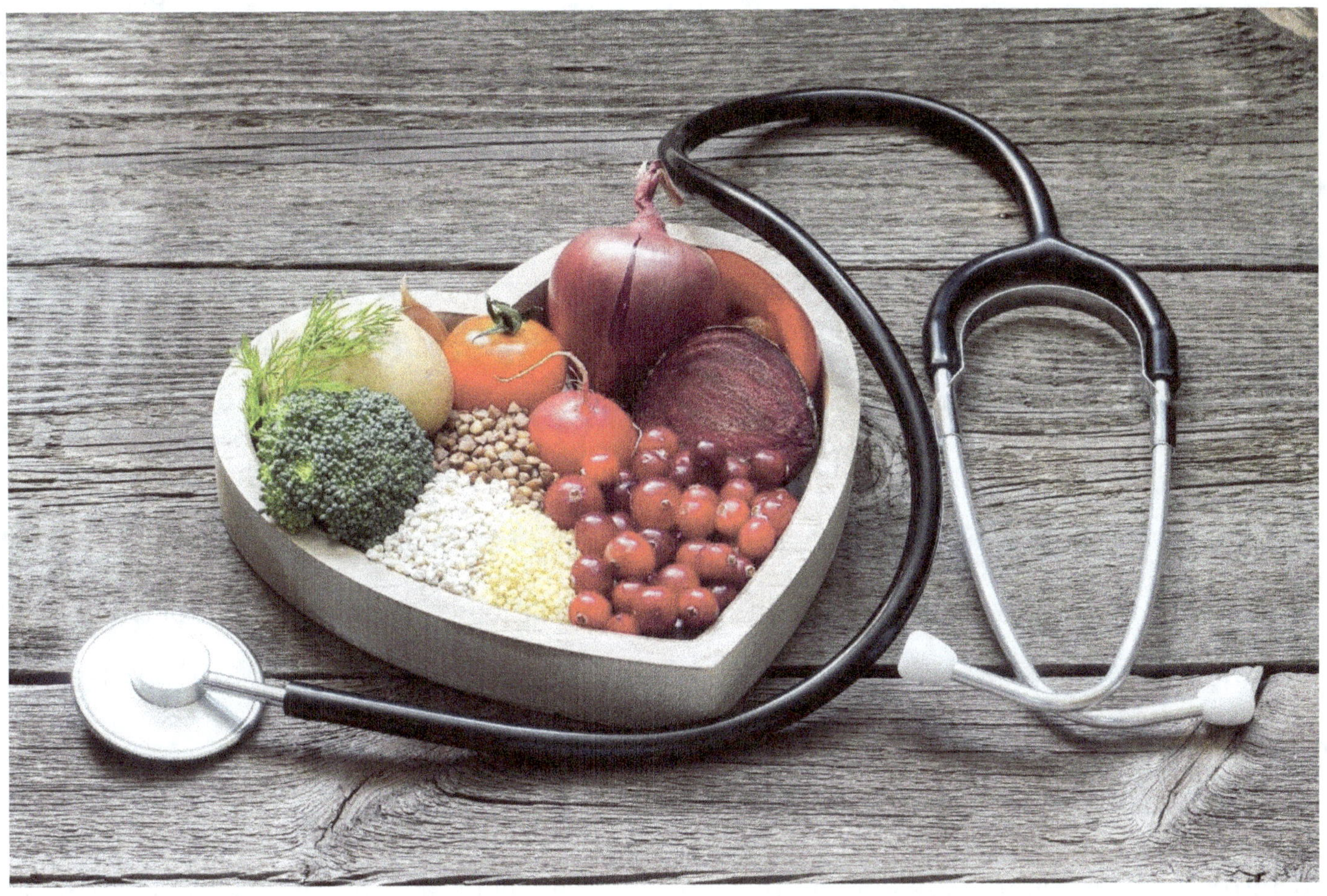

In today's world, managing diabetes effectively requires a comprehensive understanding of nutrition, lifestyle choices, and meal planning. For both men and women navigating the complexities of diabetes, making informed dietary decisions is crucial. This introduction sets the stage for a journey through the various aspects of a diabetic diet, offering practical guidance, delicious recipes, and the tools necessary to create a sustainable and enjoyable eating plan. This cookbook aims to empower individuals with diabetes to take control of their health through informed dietary choices.

The diabetic diet is not merely about restriction; it is an opportunity to embrace a wide array of foods that support overall well-being. Low-carb diabetic meal plans play a pivotal role in managing blood sugar levels, providing a foundation for individuals seeking to regulate their glucose effectively. By understanding the principles of carbohydrate counting, readers will learn to navigate food options confidently, making choices that align with their health goals. The focus will be on whole, nutrient-dense foods that not only satisfy hunger but also provide essential vitamins and minerals.

In addition to traditional meal planning, this cookbook emphasizes the significance of plant-based diets for diabetes management. Incorporating more fruits, vegetables, whole grains, legumes, and nuts can provide health benefits beyond blood sugar control. The Mediterranean diet, known for its heart-healthy properties, is also explored as a viable option for diabetics. With its emphasis on healthy fats, lean proteins, and fiber-rich foods, this dietary approach offers a flavorful and diverse array of meals that promote overall health while accommodating the specific needs of individuals with diabetes.

Snacking can often pose challenges for those managing diabetes, yet it presents an opportunity to introduce diabetic-friendly options that are both satisfying and nutritious. This cookbook includes a variety of snack ideas that are low in sugar and high in fiber, ensuring that individuals can enjoy their favorite treats without compromising their health. Additionally, gluten-free diabetic recipes will be provided to cater to those with gluten sensitivities, demonstrating that dietary restrictions do not have to limit culinary creativity.

Finally, the integration of intermittent fasting as a strategic approach to diabetes control is examined, highlighting its potential benefits for blood sugar management. Meal prep strategies will also be outlined to help individuals plan their weekly meals efficiently, reducing the likelihood of impulsive eating decisions.

From diabetes-friendly desserts to culturally specific diets, this cookbook is designed to be a comprehensive resource for anyone seeking to improve their health through nutrition. With a focus on balance and enjoyment, readers are invited to embark on a rewarding culinary journey toward better diabetes management.

Chapter 1:
Understanding Diabetes and Nutrition

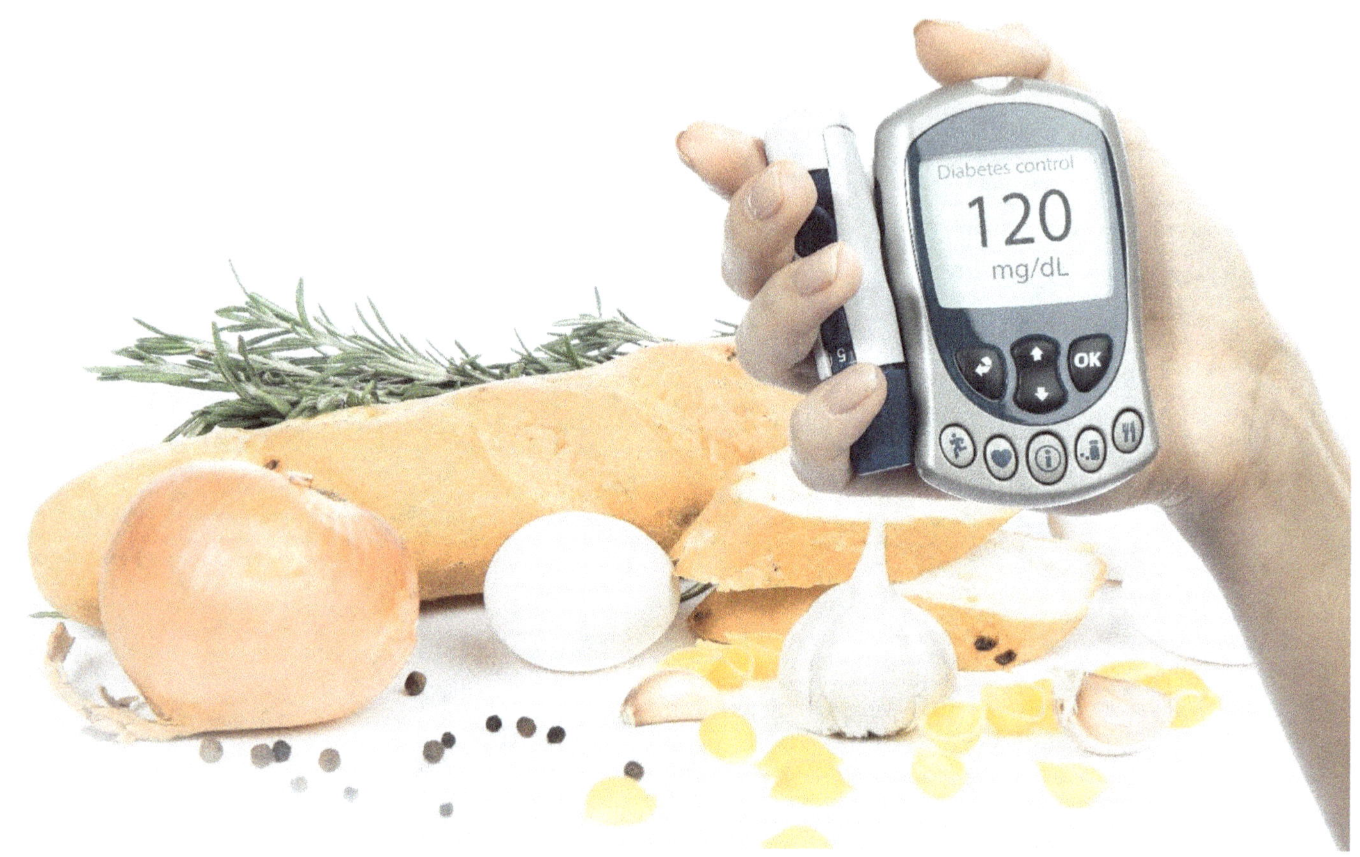

The Role of Diet in Diabetes Management

Diet plays a crucial role in the management of diabetes, influencing blood sugar levels, weight, and overall health. For individuals living with diabetes, understanding the impact of various food choices on their condition is essential. A well-structured diet helps regulate glucose levels, reduces the risk of complications, and promotes better overall well-being. This subchapter will explore various dietary approaches, including low-carb meal plans, plant-based diets, and the Mediterranean diet, each offering unique benefits for diabetes management.

Low-carb diabetic meal plans are often recommended due to their effectiveness in stabilizing blood sugar levels. By limiting carbohydrate intake, individuals can reduce the frequency and severity of glucose spikes. Foods such as non-starchy vegetables, lean proteins, and healthy fats become staples in this approach. A focus on low-carb options not only aids in blood sugar control but also assists in weight management, which is especially important for those with type 2 diabetes. Emphasizing whole foods while avoiding processed carbohydrates can lead to significant improvements in health metrics.

Plant-based diets have gained popularity as a sustainable approach to diabetes management. This diet emphasizes whole, unprocessed foods derived from plants, including fruits, vegetables, legumes, and whole grains. These foods are rich in fiber, vitamins, and minerals while being low in unhealthy fats and calories. The high fiber content of plant-based foods helps regulate blood sugar and promotes satiety, which can aid in weight control. Moreover, this dietary approach encourages the consumption of antioxidant-rich foods that may reduce inflammation and lower the risk of diabetes-related complications.

The Mediterranean diet is another effective dietary pattern for individuals with diabetes. Rich in healthy fats, particularly from olive oil, nuts, and fish, this diet emphasizes whole grains, vegetables, fruits, and legumes. Research has shown that the Mediterranean diet can improve glycemic control and cardiovascular health, making it an excellent choice for diabetics.
This diet encourages a balanced intake of macronutrients and promotes the consumption of foods that are both nutritious and satisfying. Additionally, the Mediterranean diet is versatile and can be adapted to include culturally specific foods, making it accessible to a wide range of individuals.

Incorporating diabetes-friendly snack options into daily routines can significantly enhance dietary adherence and blood sugar control. Choosing snacks that are high in protein and fiber, such as nuts, seeds, and vegetables with hummus, can help in maintaining stable blood sugar levels. These snacks can prevent excessive hunger and reduce the likelihood of overeating during meals. Moreover, gluten-free diabetic recipes cater to those with gluten sensitivities, ensuring that all individuals can enjoy satisfying and healthful options. Lastly, the consideration of intermittent fasting can also play a role in blood sugar management, as it encourages mindful eating and can help improve insulin sensitivity.

In summary, the role of diet in diabetes management cannot be overstated. By adopting a structured approach that incorporates low-carb meal plans, plant-based foods, and the Mediterranean diet, individuals can experience improved health outcomes. Furthermore, being mindful of snacking habits and exploring various dietary patterns can promote better control over blood sugar levels. Individuals are encouraged to focus on whole, nutrient-dense foods while considering their personal preferences and lifestyle to create a sustainable and effective diabetes management plan.

Overview of Plant-Based Diets

Plant-based diets have gained significant attention in recent years, particularly for their potential benefits in managing diabetes. Unlike traditional diets that may emphasize meat and animal products, plant-based diets focus on whole foods derived primarily from plants. This includes fruits, vegetables, legumes, nuts, seeds, and whole grains. By prioritizing these food groups, individuals can not only improve their overall health but also help regulate blood sugar levels, making plant-based diets a favorable option for those managing diabetes.

The key to a successful plant-based diet for diabetes lies in its ability to provide essential nutrients while minimizing processed foods and added sugars. Many plant foods are rich in fiber, which can help slow the absorption of glucose into the bloodstream, aiding in better blood sugar control. Additionally, these diets are typically lower in saturated fats and calories, which can contribute to weight management—a crucial factor in diabetes care. The Mediterranean diet, often considered a model for plant-based eating, emphasizes fruits, vegetables, whole grains, and healthy fats like olive oil, providing a balanced approach that aligns well with diabetic dietary needs.

Incorporating a variety of plant-based foods can also enhance nutrient intake, offering vitamins, minerals, and antioxidants that support overall health. For diabetic individuals, the inclusion of foods such as legumes and whole grains can provide a steady source of energy without causing drastic spikes in blood glucose levels. Moreover, plant-based diets can be customized to meet individual preferences and cultural backgrounds, making it easier for people to adopt and maintain these eating patterns. This adaptability is particularly beneficial for those looking to create culturally specific diabetic diets that resonate with their culinary traditions.

Snack options in a plant-based diet can be both delicious and diabetes-friendly. Foods such as hummus with vegetable sticks, mixed nuts, or fruit smoothies made with unsweetened almond milk serve as nutritious choices that satisfy cravings without compromising blood sugar control. Additionally, gluten-free plant-based recipes are accessible for those with dietary restrictions, ensuring that everyone can enjoy a wide range of snacks and meals without the worry of gluten-related issues. Meal prep strategies that focus on plant-based ingredients can further simplify the process of managing diabetes, allowing for easy access to healthy options throughout the week.

Finally, the potential for incorporating intermittent fasting into a plant-based eating plan offers another layer of flexibility for diabetes management. This approach can help improve insulin sensitivity and promote weight loss, which are vital components of diabetes control. By thoughtfully planning meals and snacks around fasting periods, individuals can maintain a balanced intake of nutrients while adhering to their dietary goals. Whether through meal prep or exploring diabetic-friendly desserts made from whole plant ingredients, the emphasis on plant-based eating can significantly enhance the quality of life for those managing diabetes.

Chapter 2:
The Plant-Powered Approach

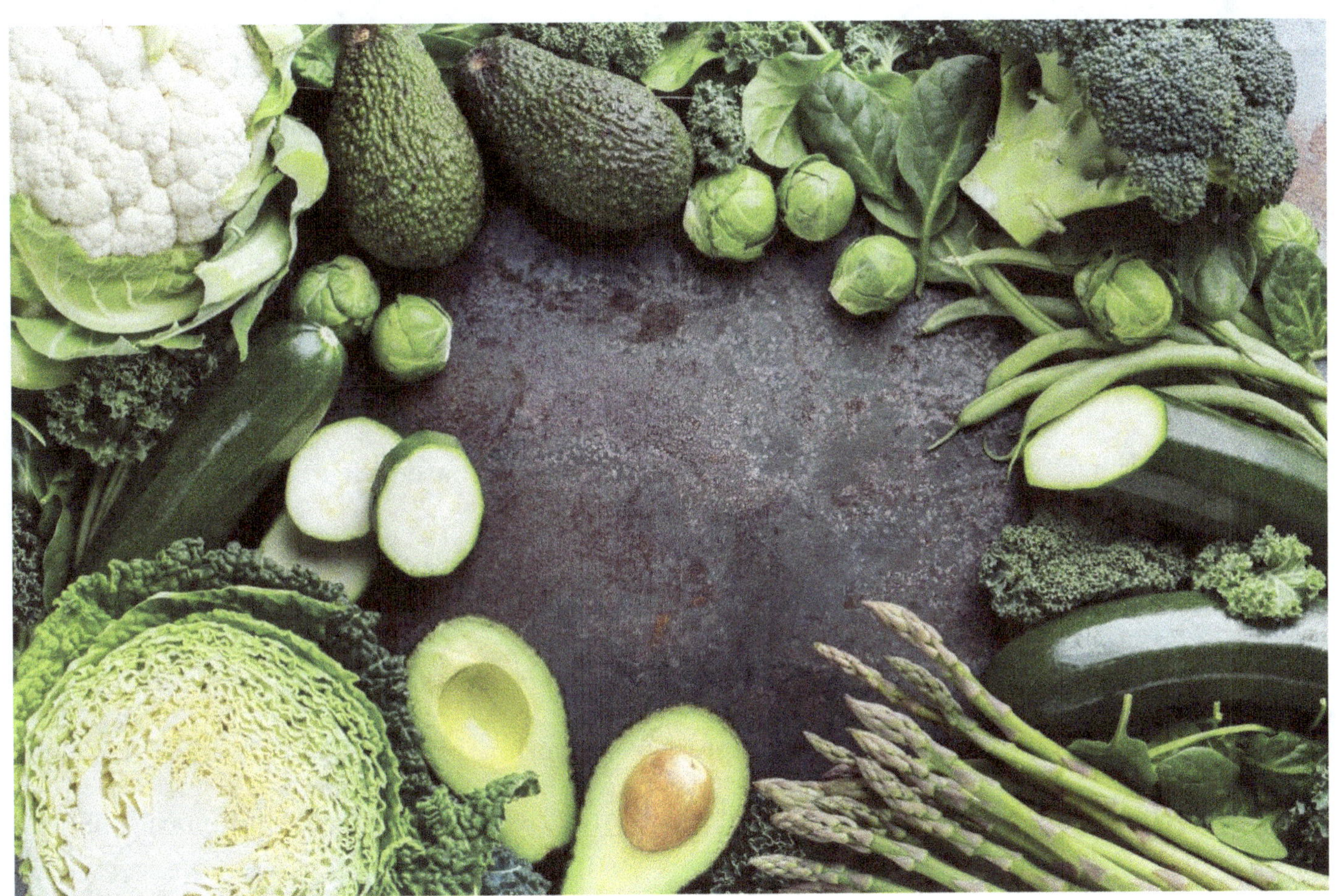

Benefits of a Plant-Based Diet

Adopting a plant-based diet offers numerous benefits for individuals managing diabetes. One of the primary advantages is its potential to improve blood sugar control. Plant-based foods are typically high in fiber, which aids in slowing down the absorption of glucose in the bloodstream.

This improved glycemic control is crucial for diabetics, as it helps prevent spikes in blood sugar levels. By focusing on whole grains, legumes, fruits, and vegetables, individuals can create meals that promote stable blood sugar levels and reduce the risk of complications associated with diabetes.

In addition to blood sugar management, a plant-based diet can support weight loss and maintenance, which are vital for people with diabetes. Many plant-based foods are lower in calories and fat compared to animal products, making it easier to achieve and maintain a healthy weight. This aspect is particularly important since excess weight can lead to insulin resistance and further complicate diabetes management. By incorporating nutrient-dense, low-calorie foods into their diets, individuals can feel satisfied while working toward their weight goals.

Cardiovascular health is another significant benefit of a plant-based diet, especially relevant for those with diabetes, who are at an increased risk of heart disease. Plant-based diets are rich in antioxidants, healthy fats, and essential nutrients that contribute to heart health. Foods such as nuts, seeds, and olive oil, commonly found in Mediterranean diets, provide healthy fats that can improve cholesterol levels and lower blood pressure. By prioritizing these foods, individuals can enhance their overall cardiovascular health, reducing the risk of heart-related complications.

Moreover, the anti-inflammatory properties of a plant-based diet can play a crucial role in diabetes management. Chronic inflammation is often linked to insulin resistance and other complications associated with diabetes. By consuming a variety of fruits, vegetables, whole grains, and legumes, individuals can benefit from an array of phytonutrients that combat inflammation. This dietary approach not only helps in managing diabetes but also promotes overall well-being, enhancing the quality of life for those living with the condition.

Lastly, a plant-based diet can encourage creativity and variety in meal planning, making it easier to adhere to dietary guidelines. With a wide range of foods to choose from, individuals can explore diverse cuisines and flavors, ensuring that meals remain enjoyable and satisfying.

Incorporating culturally specific foods and recipes can also foster a sense of connection and community, which is essential for maintaining motivation in managing diabetes. By embracing a plant-based approach, individuals can create delicious, diabetic-friendly meals that support their health goals while enjoying the process of cooking and eating.

Essential Nutrients for Diabetics

Essential nutrients play a crucial role in managing diabetes effectively, ensuring that individuals can maintain stable blood glucose levels while enjoying a varied and satisfying diet. For both men and women with diabetes, understanding the significance of these nutrients can empower them to make informed dietary choices that support their overall health. Key nutrients include carbohydrates, proteins, fats, vitamins, and minerals, each contributing to a balanced diet that promotes better glycemic control and reduces the risk of complications associated with diabetes.

Carbohydrates, while often viewed with caution by diabetics, are essential for energy. The focus should be on selecting complex carbohydrates that have a low glycemic index, such as whole grains, legumes, and vegetables. These foods release glucose slowly into the bloodstream, preventing spikes in blood sugar levels. Additionally, incorporating fiber-rich foods can enhance satiety and aid in digestion, making it easier for individuals to manage their weight and blood sugar levels effectively.

Proteins also play an important role in a diabetic diet. They help to build and repair tissues, support immune function, and can contribute to the feeling of fullness, which is beneficial for weight management. Lean sources of protein, such as chicken, turkey, fish, beans, and legumes, are particularly advantageous. For those following specific dietary patterns, such as plant-based or Mediterranean diets, it is essential to include a variety of protein sources to ensure adequate intake of essential amino acids while minimizing saturated fats.

Healthy fats are another crucial nutrient for diabetics. They help to promote heart health, which is vital since individuals with diabetes are at a higher risk for cardiovascular diseases. Unsaturated fats, found in olive oil, avocados, nuts, and seeds, should be prioritized over saturated and trans fats. Including these fats in moderation can enhance the flavor of meals while contributing to overall health. Furthermore, omega-3 fatty acids, found in fatty fish and flaxseeds, have been shown to have anti-inflammatory properties, which can be beneficial for those managing diabetes.

Lastly, vitamins and minerals are essential for various bodily functions, including immune support and energy production. A well-rounded diet rich in fruits, vegetables, whole grains, and lean proteins can help ensure that individuals receive adequate amounts of these micronutrients.

In some cases, nutritional supplements may be necessary to fill gaps in the diet, especially for those following restrictive diets. Consulting with a healthcare provider or dietitian can help determine individual needs and ensure a balanced intake of essential nutrients, ultimately aiding in the management of diabetes and enhancing overall health.

How to Transition to a Plant-Based Diet

Transitioning to a plant-based diet can be a rewarding journey, particularly for individuals managing diabetes. This dietary approach emphasizes whole foods derived from plants, including fruits, vegetables, legumes, nuts, and seeds, while minimizing or eliminating animal products. For those with diabetes, a plant-based diet can provide an array of health benefits, such as improved blood sugar control, reduced cholesterol levels, and enhanced weight management. The key to a successful transition lies in understanding the principles of plant-based eating and integrating them gradually into your daily routine.

To begin the transition, start by incorporating more plant-based meals into your weekly menu. This can be as simple as replacing one or two meat-based meals with plant-based alternatives. For instance, try a lentil stew or a chickpea salad instead of a traditional meat dish. Gradually increasing the proportion of plant-based foods will help your palate adjust while also allowing you to explore new flavors and textures. Additionally, consider adopting a Mediterranean approach, which emphasizes healthy fats from sources like olive oil and nuts, along with a variety of fruits and vegetables. This combination not only supports diabetes management but also enhances overall well-being.

Meal planning is essential for a successful transition to a plant-based diet, particularly for those managing diabetes. Create a weekly meal plan that includes a diverse range of plant-based recipes, ensuring that you meet your nutritional needs while keeping blood sugar levels stable. Focus on low-carb options, such as zucchini noodles, cauliflower rice, and leafy greens, which can help control insulin responses. Preparing meals in advance can also save time and reduce stress during busy weekdays, making it easier to stick to your dietary goals.

As you explore plant-based eating, it's vital to ensure you're receiving adequate nutrients, particularly protein and essential vitamins. Incorporate a variety of legumes, whole grains, nuts, and seeds into your meals to obtain the necessary nutrients. This strategy not only supports blood sugar control but also promotes a balanced diet. Additionally, consider nutritional supplements if needed, to fill any gaps in your diet. Consulting with a healthcare professional or a registered dietitian can provide personalized guidance and help you navigate potential deficiencies.

Lastly, consider the role of snacks in your plant-based diet. Opt for diabetic-friendly snacks such as vegetable sticks with hummus, mixed nuts, or fruit with nut butter. These options are not only delicious but also align with your dietary goals. By focusing on whole, minimally processed foods, you'll find that your energy levels improve and cravings diminish. The transition to a plant-based diet may take time, but with careful planning and patience, you can create a sustainable eating pattern that supports your diabetes management and overall health.

Chapter 3:
Affordable Recipes for Beginners

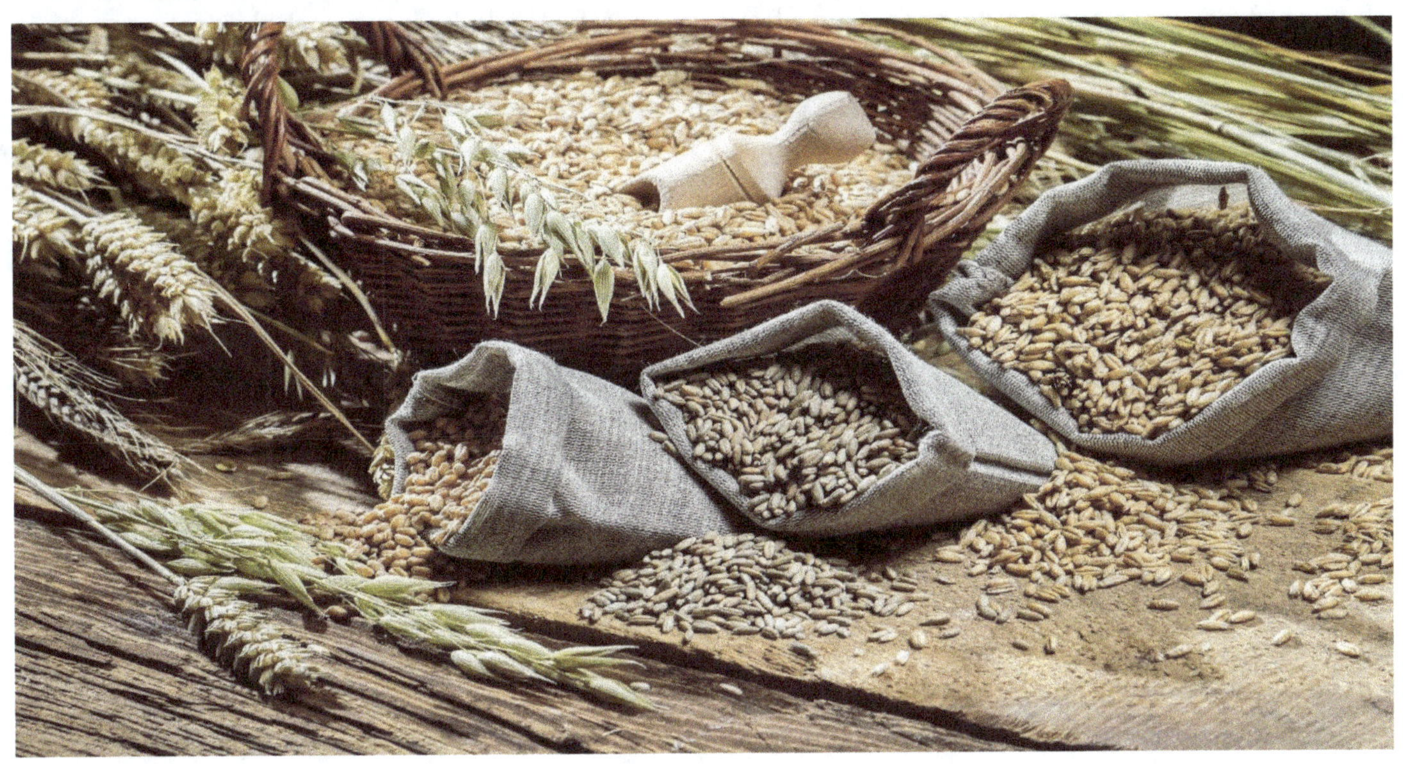

Simple Ingredients, Big Flavor

In the realm of diabetic cooking, the notion that simple ingredients can yield big flavors is a principle that holds significant value. Many individuals managing diabetes may feel overwhelmed by the limitations often associated with dietary restrictions. However, embracing the philosophy of utilizing uncomplicated, fresh ingredients can transform meals into delightful culinary experiences without sacrificing taste or nutritional integrity. Focusing on whole foods, such as vegetables, lean proteins, whole grains, and healthy fats, not only supports blood sugar management but also enhances overall well-being.

Utilizing herbs and spices is a key strategy for maximizing flavor while keeping ingredients simple. Fresh herbs like basil, cilantro, and parsley can elevate a dish, adding depth and complexity without the need for excessive salt or fat. Similarly, spices such as cumin, turmeric, and paprika can introduce warmth and richness to meals. These flavor-enhancing elements are particularly beneficial for those following a low-carb or Mediterranean diet, as they encourage the use of natural flavors over processed alternatives, effectively keeping carbohydrate counts in check while delivering satisfying meals.

Incorporating plant-based ingredients into a diabetic diet can also contribute to vibrant flavors that are both nutritious and satisfying. Using seasonal vegetables not only supports local agriculture but also ensures that meals are bursting with freshness. For instance, roasted bell peppers, zucchini, and eggplant can serve as a base for various dishes, infusing them with sweetness and texture. When paired with legumes or whole grains, these ingredients create balanced, flavorful meals suitable for anyone managing diabetes, including those following gluten-free or culturally specific diets.

Snacking can pose challenges for individuals on a diabetic diet, but it can also be an opportunity to embrace simple ingredients that pack a flavorful punch. Options such as hummus made from chickpeas or guacamole with ripe avocados provide nutritious, satisfying snacks that are low in carbohydrates. Pairing these dips with fresh vegetables or whole-grain crackers allows for a satisfying crunch while keeping blood sugar levels stable. By focusing on easy-to-prepare snacks, individuals can maintain energy levels and curb cravings without resorting to processed, high-sugar alternatives.

Meal prep strategies play a crucial role in successfully navigating a diabetic diet while maximizing flavor. Planning meals ahead of time allows for better control over ingredient choices and portion sizes. Preparing versatile components, such as grilled chicken, quinoa, or mixed roasted vegetables, can create a solid foundation for various meals throughout the week. By keeping flavors simple yet bold, individuals can enjoy a diverse range of dishes, from salads to soups, ensuring that adhering to dietary guidelines remains a rewarding and enjoyable experience.

One-Pot Meals for Easy Cleanup

One-pot meals offer a practical solution for those managing diabetes while minimizing cleanup. These meals simplify the cooking process, allowing individuals to focus on nourishing their bodies without the hassle of multiple dishes. By integrating various food groups into a single pot, one can create balanced meals that align with diabetic dietary needs. The convenience of one-pot cooking also encourages home meal preparation, which is essential for controlling carbohydrate intake and managing blood sugar levels effectively.

When planning one-pot meals, consider utilizing lean proteins such as chicken, turkey, or plant-based sources like lentils and chickpeas. These ingredients provide essential nutrients while keeping the carbohydrate count low. Incorporating a variety of vegetables not only enhances flavor but also adds fiber, which is beneficial for digestion and helps regulate blood sugar levels. Opt for seasonal produce to ensure freshness and maximize nutritional value. This diverse combination of ingredients can help create satisfying meals that comply with diabetic dietary guidelines.

Herbs and spices are vital in transforming one-pot meals into flavorful dishes without the need for added sugars or unhealthy fats. Consider Mediterranean-inspired recipes that utilize olive oil, garlic, and herbs like oregano and basil. These ingredients not only complement the flavors of the dish but also contribute to heart health, which is particularly important for individuals with diabetes. Experimenting with different cuisines can introduce variety and excitement into meal planning, making it easier to adhere to dietary restrictions.

In addition to their health benefits, one-pot meals are ideal for meal prep and batch cooking. Preparing larger quantities allows for leftovers, making it easier to stick to a consistent eating schedule, particularly for those practicing intermittent fasting. Leftovers can be portioned and stored for future meals, ensuring that nutritious options are readily available during busy weekdays. This strategy not only saves time but also reinforces healthy eating habits, essential for effective diabetes management.

Lastly, one-pot meals can be easily adapted to accommodate specific dietary needs, such as gluten-free or culturally specific diets. By selecting appropriate grains or substituting ingredients, these meals can cater to a wide range of preferences and requirements.

This flexibility makes one-pot cooking a viable option for everyone, ensuring that managing diabetes does not mean sacrificing flavor or variety in one's diet. Embracing one-pot meals can lead to a more enjoyable cooking experience while promoting healthier eating habits essential for diabetes control.

Budget-Friendly Pantry Staples

In managing diabetes, maintaining a well-stocked pantry with budget-friendly staples can significantly ease meal preparation while adhering to dietary guidelines. These staples not only support a low-carb approach but also align with various dietary preferences, including plant-based and Mediterranean diets. By focusing on budget-friendly ingredients, individuals can create wholesome meals without compromising on nutrition or flavor. Essential items such as whole grains, legumes, and canned vegetables serve as the foundation for balanced meals, making them accessible for everyone.

Whole grains, such as brown rice, quinoa, and barley, provide valuable fiber and nutrients while being versatile enough to complement various dishes. They can be used as a base for salads, stir-fries, or as side dishes. Incorporating whole grains into a diabetic diet helps regulate blood sugar levels while ensuring satiety. In addition to being budget-friendly, these grains are easy to prepare in bulk, allowing for efficient meal prep strategies that cater to busy lifestyles.

Legumes, including lentils, chickpeas, and black beans, are another essential pantry staple. They are not only affordable but also rich in protein and fiber, making them an excellent choice for those following a plant-based diet. Legumes can be added to soups, salads, and stews, contributing both texture and nutritional value. Their high fiber content supports digestive health and helps stabilize blood sugar levels, making them a smart addition for diabetes management.

Canned vegetables and fruits, particularly those without added sugars or sodium, are incredibly convenient and cost-effective. They provide essential vitamins and minerals, making it easy to incorporate a variety of nutrients into meals. Items like canned tomatoes, green beans, and low-sodium corn can enhance soups and sauces, while canned fruits can serve as healthy snacks or dessert options when fresh produce is not available. When selecting canned goods, it's important to read labels carefully to ensure they fit within a diabetic-friendly dietary framework.

Finally, incorporating herbs, spices, and healthy oils into the pantry can elevate the flavor of meals without adding unnecessary carbohydrates. Items like olive oil, vinegar, garlic, and various dried herbs not only enhance taste but also provide health benefits associated with the Mediterranean diet. By focusing on these budget-friendly pantry staples, individuals can prepare flavorful, nutritious meals that support diabetes management while adhering to personal dietary preferences.

Chapter 4:
Quick and Easy Diabetic Recipes

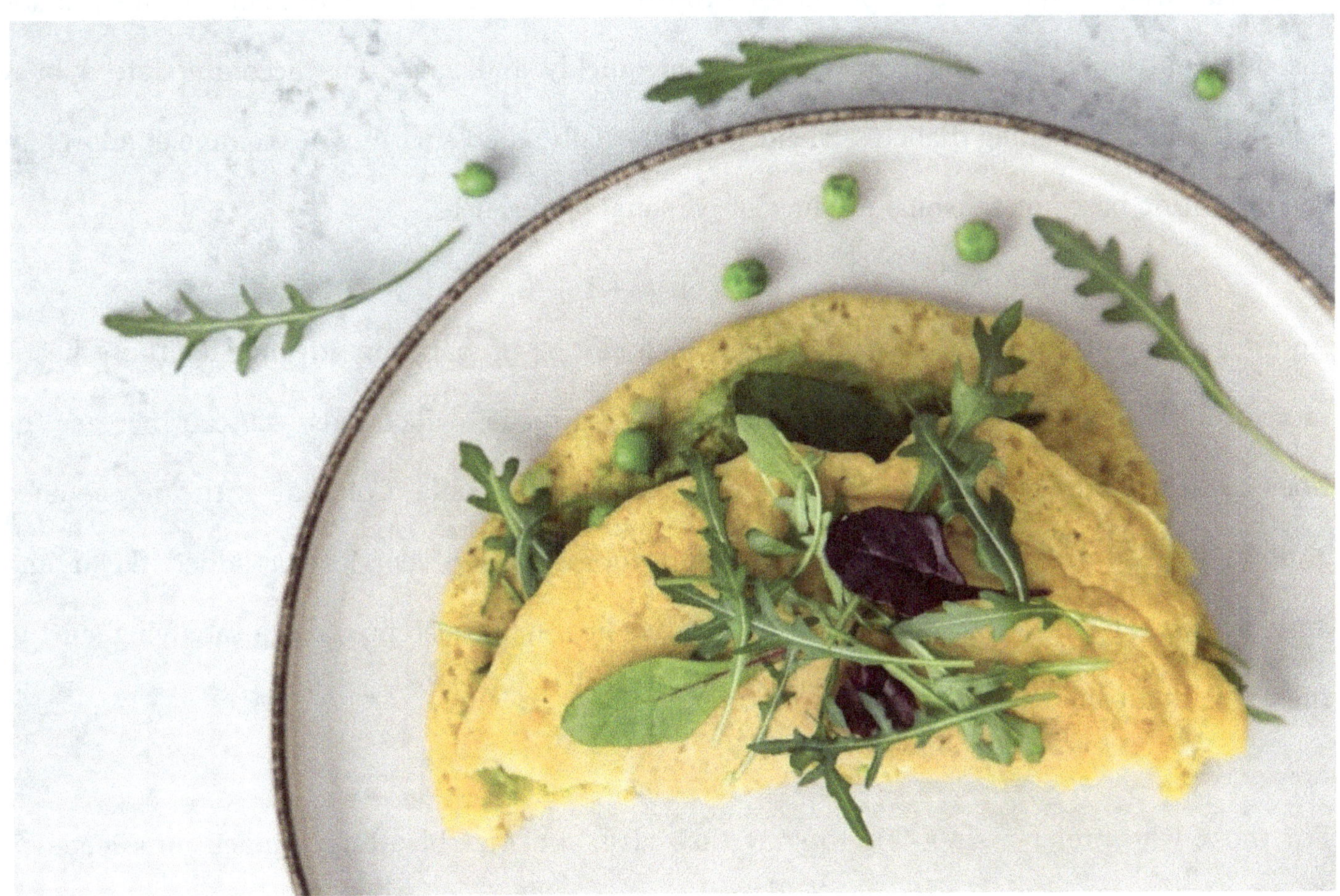

Breakfast Ideas

Breakfast is often referred to as the most important meal of the day, and for individuals managing diabetes, it takes on added significance. A well-balanced breakfast can set the tone for the rest of the day, helping to stabilize blood sugar levels while providing essential nutrients.

When planning breakfast options, it's crucial to focus on low-carb ingredients that are rich in fiber, protein, and healthy fats. This not only supports effective weight management but also ensures a steady release of energy throughout the morning.

One simple yet effective breakfast idea is a chickpea omelet. Using a variety of non-starchy vegetables such as spinach, bell peppers, and tomatoes, you can create a colorful and nutritious meal. Pair this with a side of avocado for healthy fats, which can enhance satiety and provide essential nutrients. This dish can be prepared quickly and can easily accommodate a busy schedule while remaining diabetes-friendly. Additionally, the versatility of the omelet allows for customization based on seasonal produce or personal preferences.

Another excellent option is overnight oats, which can be prepared in advance for those hectic mornings. By using rolled oats and incorporating chia seeds or flaxseeds, you can increase the fiber content while keeping the carbohydrate count manageable. Combine with unsweetened almond milk, a scoop of protein powder, and your choice of berries for added flavor and antioxidants. This meal not only supports digestive health but also provides a satisfying start to the day without spiking blood sugar levels.

For those who prefer a smoothie to start their day, consider blending spinach, unsweetened Greek yogurt, a small portion of fruit, and unsweetened almond milk. This combination delivers a refreshing and nutrient-rich breakfast option. The protein from Greek yogurt helps maintain blood sugar levels, while the fiber from spinach and fruit ensures a feeling of fullness. Smoothies can also be a convenient way to incorporate more plant-based ingredients, making them suitable for those exploring diabetic-friendly vegan options.

Lastly, whole grain toast topped with nut butter and slices of banana or strawberries presents another quick and satisfying breakfast choice. Opt for whole grain or sprouted bread to maximize fiber intake, and choose natural nut butter without added sugars. The healthy fats and protein from the nut butter, combined with the natural sweetness of fruit, create a balanced meal that sustains energy levels. This option is not only easy to prepare but also provides the comfort and satisfaction often sought in breakfast foods, making it a perfect fit for busy families.

Lunch Solutions

When it comes to lunch, finding meals that are both satisfying and suitable for a diabetic diet can be a challenge, especially for busy families. The key to creating effective lunch solutions lies in focusing on balanced nutrition while ensuring preparation is quick and straightforward. Incorporating lean proteins, healthy fats, and whole grains can not only help manage blood sugar levels but also keep energy levels stable throughout the day. By planning ahead and utilizing simple recipes, families can enjoy delicious meals without the stress.

One-pot meals serve as an excellent option for lunchtime, providing a convenient way to combine various food groups into a single dish. Consider a quinoa and black bean bowl, which packs protein, fiber, and essential nutrients into a colorful and filling meal. The versatility of ingredients allows for adjustments based on seasonal availability or personal preferences, making it easy to keep meals interesting. Additionally, these one-pot creations often yield leftovers, providing an effortless solution for the next day's lunch.

For those seeking a lighter option, salads can be a refreshing and nutritious choice. Starting with a base of leafy greens, adding lean proteins such as grilled chicken or chickpeas, and tossing in a variety of vegetables creates a satisfying meal.

Drizzling with a homemade vinaigrette not only enhances flavor but allows for control over sugar and calorie content. Salads can be customized to reflect personal tastes and dietary needs, ensuring that each family member finds something they enjoy.

Incorporating international flavors can also enhance lunch options. Dishes like a Mediterranean wrap filled with hummus, cucumber, tomatoes, and grilled chicken offer a healthy twist on traditional favorites. Alternatively, a vegetable stir-fry with tofu and a light soy sauce can provide a quick and fulfilling meal. Exploring global cuisines not only adds variety but also introduces new ingredients that can support a balanced diabetic diet, making lunchtime more exciting and enjoyable.

Finally, smoothies and beverages can serve as both a meal replacement and a refreshing addition to lunch. A spinach and berry smoothie, blended with unsweetened almond milk, provides essential vitamins and minerals while being low in carbohydrates. This option is particularly appealing for those on the go, as it can be prepared in advance and taken anywhere. By integrating these diverse options into your lunch routine, families can ensure they are eating healthily while managing diabetes effectively.

Dinner Delights

Dinner is often the centerpiece of family life, a time to gather and enjoy a meal together after a long day. For those managing diabetes, preparing satisfying dinners that align with dietary needs can be a challenge. In this section, we will explore a variety of dinner delights that are not only quick and easy to prepare but also cater to the diverse requirements of a diabetic diet. Each recipe is designed to be flavorful, nourishing, and suitable for busy families seeking to maintain a healthy lifestyle.

One-pot meals are an excellent option for those who want to minimize cleanup while still serving a nutritious dinner. These recipes typically combine protein, vegetables, and whole grains or legumes, allowing for a balanced meal in one dish. For instance, a savory chicken and vegetable stew can be prepared in under 30 minutes using a slow cooker or stovetop. This method not only saves time but also ensures that the flavors meld beautifully, creating a comforting dish that everyone will enjoy.

For families looking to incorporate more plant-based options, consider recipes that feature nutrient-dense ingredients such as lentils, quinoa, and a variety of vegetables. A hearty vegetable stir-fry with tofu can serve as a delightful main course while providing essential nutrients and protein. This dish can be customized with seasonal vegetables to enhance freshness and flavor. Plant-based meals are often lower in carbohydrates and can aid in weight management, making them an ideal choice for diabetic-friendly cooking.

Comfort foods need not be off-limits for those managing diabetes. By making simple substitutions, traditional favorites can be adapted to fit a diabetic diet. For example, instead of creamy pasta dishes, consider using whole grain or legume-based pasta and pairing it with a homemade tomato sauce loaded with fresh herbs and vegetables. These adjustments not only retain the comforting essence of the original dish but also contribute to better blood sugar control.

Finally, no dinner is complete without a satisfying dessert or snack. Diabetic-friendly options can still be indulgent without compromising health. Consider creating a fruit-based dessert, such as baked apples with cinnamon and a sprinkle of nuts, which delivers natural sweetness and fiber. Alternatively, smoothies made with low-fat yogurt, fresh fruits, and spinach can serve as a delicious and nutritious way to end a meal. These recipes highlight that it is possible to enjoy delightful dinners while adhering to dietary guidelines, making mealtime a pleasure for the entire family.

Snack Options

When it comes to managing diabetes, choosing the right snacks can play an essential role in maintaining stable blood sugar levels while satisfying hunger between meals. The key is to focus on options that are low in refined carbohydrates and added sugars, yet high in nutrients. This subchapter presents a variety of snack ideas that are not only diabetes-friendly but also quick and easy to prepare, making them ideal for busy families.

One great option is fresh vegetables paired with a healthy dip. Carrot sticks, cucumber slices, and bell pepper strips can be cut ahead of time and stored in the refrigerator for easy access. Pair these veggies with hummus or a Greek yogurt-based dip for added flavor and protein. This combination provides fiber and essential vitamins while keeping carbohydrate intake in check, making it a perfect choice for a mid-afternoon snack.

Another delicious and satisfying snack option is a small handful of nuts. Almonds, walnuts, or pistachios are excellent choices due to their healthy fat content and ability to promote satiety. They can be portioned out into small containers or bags for on-the-go convenience. Just be mindful of portion sizes, as nuts are calorie-dense. A serving of about 1 ounce can provide a satisfying crunch without the blood sugar spikes associated with more traditional snack foods.

For those with a sweet tooth, consider fresh fruit or a small serving of berries. Fruits such as apples, pears, or berries offer natural sweetness along with important nutrients and fiber.

Pairing fruit with a source of protein, such as a slice of low-fat cheese or a small dollop of nut butter, can further help to stabilize blood sugar levels. This combination not only satisfies cravings but also provides a well-rounded snack option that fits within a diabetic dietary framework.

Lastly, consider preparing simple homemade snacks that can be made in batch and stored for later use. Energy balls made from oats, nut butter, and seeds are a nutritious option that can be customized with various flavors and ingredients. Another idea is to create baked kale chips or roasted chickpeas, which offer a crunchy alternative to traditional snacks. These homemade options allow for control over ingredients and can be tailored to suit individual taste preferences, ensuring that healthy snacking is both enjoyable and accessible.

Chapter 5:
Low-Carb Diabetic Meal Plans

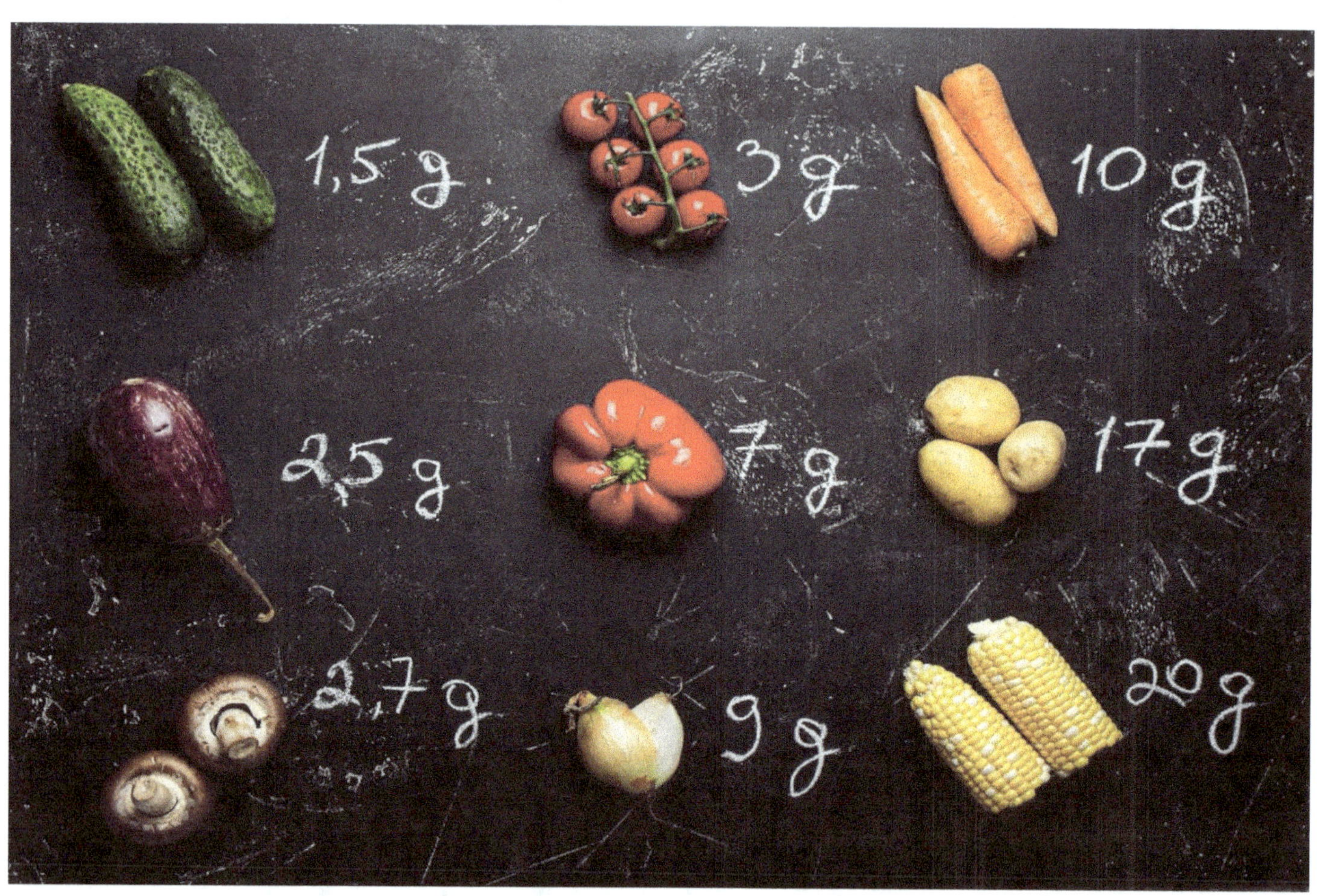

Introduction to Low-Carb Diets

Low-carb diets have gained significant traction in the realm of diabetes management, offering an effective approach to regulate blood sugar levels while still providing satisfying meal options. For individuals with diabetes, managing carbohydrate intake is crucial, as carbohydrates have a direct impact on blood glucose levels.

This subchapter will introduce the principles of low-carb diets, their benefits for diabetics, and how they can be adapted to fit various dietary preferences, including plant-based and Mediterranean approaches.

At its core, a low-carb diet emphasizes the reduction of carbohydrate intake, which can lead to improved glycemic control and weight management. By limiting carbohydrates, the body is encouraged to utilize fat as a primary source of energy, a process known as ketosis. This shift not only aids in stabilizing blood sugar levels but may also result in decreased hunger and cravings, making it easier for individuals to adhere to their meal plans. For those with diabetes, achieving and maintaining a healthy weight is essential, and a low-carb diet can serve as a powerful tool in this endeavor.

Incorporating low-carb principles does not mean sacrificing flavor or nutrition. Many people are surprised to find that a variety of delicious foods can be included in their daily meals. From fresh vegetables and lean proteins to healthy fats, the options are abundant. Furthermore, low-carb diets can be tailored to accommodate specific dietary needs, such as gluten-free requirements or preferences for plant-based diets. This adaptability makes low-carb eating accessible and enjoyable for a broad audience, ensuring that individuals can find meals that suit their taste and lifestyle.

The Mediterranean diet, known for its health benefits, can also align with low-carb principles, offering a rich array of ingredients that support diabetes management. With an emphasis on whole foods like fruits, vegetables, legumes, nuts, healthy fats, and lean proteins, this dietary approach promotes not only heart health but also stable blood sugar levels. By focusing on quality ingredients and mindful eating, individuals can create a balanced and satisfying diet that meets their nutritional needs while effectively managing diabetes.

As we delve further into this cookbook, readers will discover a plethora of low-carb diabetic meal plans, snack ideas, and even dessert options that adhere to these dietary principles. Each recipe is designed to be both diabetic-friendly and delicious, ensuring that individuals can enjoy their meals without compromising their health. Additionally, practical strategies for meal prep and planning will be provided, empowering readers to take control of their dietary choices and navigate the complexities of managing diabetes with confidence.

Sample Low-Carb Meal Plan

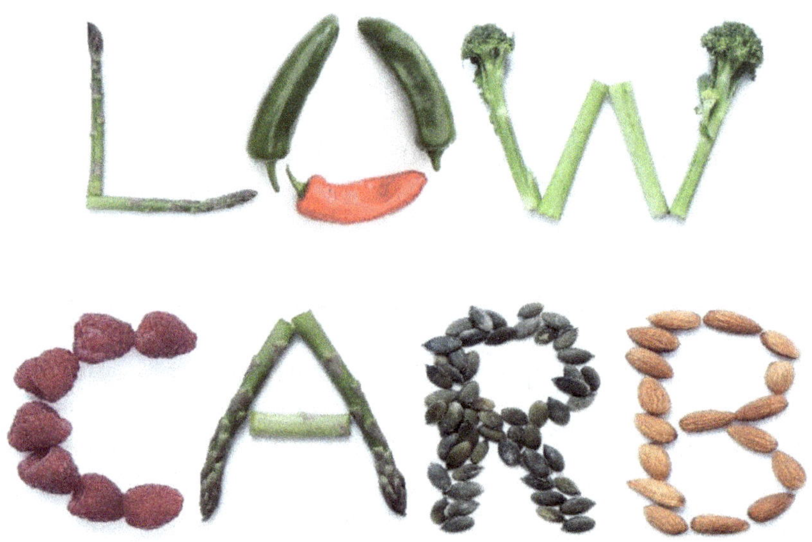

A well-structured low-carb meal plan can significantly benefit individuals managing diabetes, providing essential nutrients while stabilizing blood sugar levels. This sample meal plan incorporates diverse foods that adhere to the principles of a low-carb diet, ensuring balanced nutrition without sacrificing flavor. Each meal is designed to be diabetic-friendly, emphasizing whole, unprocessed foods that align with the Mediterranean diet and plant-based eating patterns.

For breakfast, consider a vegetable omelet made with fresh spinach, tomatoes, and bell peppers, cooked in olive oil. Pair this with a slice of gluten-free whole grain toast and a serving of avocado for healthy fats. This combination not only provides protein and fiber but also keeps carbohydrate intake low. A cup of unsweetened herbal tea or black coffee can complement this meal, enhancing your morning routine without added sugars.

Lunch can feature a hearty salad with mixed greens, cherry tomatoes, cucumbers, and grilled chicken or chickpeas for a plant-based option. Drizzle with a homemade vinaigrette made from olive oil and lemon juice to add flavor while keeping carbohydrates in check. This meal is rich in antioxidants and healthy fats, and it can be prepared in advance as part of a meal prep strategy to save time during busy weekdays.

For an afternoon snack, consider a serving of Greek yogurt topped with a handful of berries and a sprinkle of chia seeds. This snack provides protein and healthy fats while satisfying sweet cravings without causing blood sugar spikes. Alternatively, a small portion of raw vegetables such as carrot sticks or bell pepper slices with hummus can serve as a crunchy, satisfying option.

Dinner may include baked salmon seasoned with herbs, served alongside roasted Brussels sprouts and quinoa. This meal highlights the Mediterranean influence, incorporating healthy fats from the fish and fiber from the vegetables and whole grains. To finish the day, a small portion of dark chocolate or a fruit salad made with seasonal fruits can serve as a diabetic-friendly dessert, ensuring that sweet indulgences are still possible within a low-carb framework.

Tips for Low-Carb Grocery Shopping

When embarking on a low-carb grocery shopping trip, it is essential to equip yourself with a strategic approach to make informed choices that align with your dietary goals. Begin by creating a detailed shopping list that prioritizes whole, unprocessed foods.

Focus on including plenty of non-starchy vegetables, such as leafy greens, bell peppers, and broccoli, which are low in carbohydrates yet high in nutrients. Incorporating a variety of colors in your vegetable selection can also ensure a diverse nutrient intake, vital for overall health and diabetes management.

Protein sources should be a cornerstone of your shopping list. Opt for lean meats, fish, eggs, and plant-based proteins like legumes, tofu, and tempeh. When selecting packaged proteins, scrutinize labels for added sugars and carbohydrates. Additionally, consider incorporating Mediterranean diet staples such as olive oil, nuts, and seeds, which not only provide healthy fats but also contribute to satiety. These options can help sustain energy levels while managing blood sugar.

When it comes to dairy products, choose full-fat options when possible, as they usually contain fewer carbohydrates than their low-fat counterparts. Unsweetened almond milk, Greek yogurt, and cottage cheese can serve as excellent additions to your diet. Be vigilant about flavored varieties, as they often contain added sugars that can spike blood sugar levels. For those following a gluten-free diabetic diet, explore gluten-free grains like quinoa and brown rice in moderation, ensuring they fit within your overall carbohydrate goals.

Snacks are an essential component of a balanced diabetic diet, so it is prudent to stock up on diabetic-friendly snack options. Look for nuts, seeds, and low-carb protein bars that can provide quick energy without causing blood sugar fluctuations. Fresh fruits, while higher in carbs, can be enjoyed in moderation; berries, for instance, are lower in sugar and can be a delightful addition to your snack repertoire. Meal prepping can also facilitate healthy snacking—pre-portioning snacks in advance can prevent impulsive choices that may not align with your dietary requirements.

Lastly, don't overlook the importance of reading ingredient labels and being mindful of portion sizes. Many products marketed as "healthy" can still contain hidden sugars and carbs that can derail your efforts. Familiarize yourself with common alternative names for sugar and carbohydrates to ensure that you are making the best choices. By implementing these shopping tips, you can better navigate the grocery store, making informed decisions that support your low-carb diabetic meal plans and overall health.

Chapter 6:
Diabetic-Friendly Slow Cooker Recipes

Breakfast in the Slow Cooker

Breakfast can often be a challenging meal for those managing diabetes, especially when trying to balance flavor with nutritional needs. Using a slow cooker for breakfast not only simplifies meal preparation but also allows for the creation of delicious, diabetic-friendly dishes that can cater to various dietary preferences. This method enables you to set your ingredients in the evening and wake up to a warm, hearty meal, making it an excellent option for busy mornings.

One versatile ingredient that shines in slow cooker breakfasts is oats. Steel-cut oats are a great choice for a low-carb, high-fiber breakfast. When cooked overnight, they develop a creamy texture and can be flavored with spices such as cinnamon or nutmeg. Adding nuts, seeds, or a small amount of fruit can enhance the nutritional profile without significantly increasing carbohydrate content. For those following plant-based diets, using non-dairy milk can complement the oats while keeping the dish vegan-friendly.

Incorporating vegetables into breakfast can be a game changer for diabetes management. A vegetable frittata made in a slow cooker allows for a variety of colorful, nutrient-dense ingredients to be included, such as spinach, bell peppers, and tomatoes.

Eggs provide protein, which is essential for stabilizing blood sugar levels. This dish can easily be adapted to suit Mediterranean diet principles by adding ingredients like feta cheese or olives, offering a savory start to the day that aligns with healthy eating patterns.

Another delightful option for slow cooker breakfast is a quinoa porridge. Quinoa is a complete protein and contains a lower glycemic index compared to traditional grains, making it a smart choice for those with diabetes. Cooked with almond milk and spiced with vanilla and cinnamon, this porridge can be topped with fresh berries or a sprinkle of nuts for added texture and flavor. This dish not only supports a gluten-free lifestyle but also fits seamlessly into a broader diabetic meal plan.

Finally, incorporating intermittent fasting principles can be facilitated by preparing breakfast in the slow cooker. You can prepare your meal to be ready just before your eating window opens, ensuring a nutritious start to your day without the hassle of morning cooking. Additionally, meal prep strategies can be enhanced by using the slow cooker to prepare multiple portions of breakfast, allowing for easy reheating throughout the week. This approach not only saves time but also ensures that healthy, diabetic-friendly options are readily available, supporting overall dietary goals.

Hearty Soups and Stews

Hearty soups and stews offer a comforting solution for individuals managing diabetes while still craving flavorful and satisfying meals. These dishes can be tailored to align with various dietary preferences and restrictions, making them versatile options for anyone following a diabetic diet. When prepared with low-carb ingredients, these meals can help regulate blood sugar levels while providing essential nutrients, warmth, and satisfaction.

Utilizing fresh vegetables, lean proteins, and healthy fats, hearty soups and stews not only promote wellness but also serve as a nourishing staple in a balanced meal plan.

Incorporating legumes, such as lentils and beans, into soups and stews can enhance their nutritional profile while keeping carbohydrate content in check. These ingredients are high in fiber and protein, aiding in blood sugar management and promoting satiety. For those interested in a plant-based approach, consider using vegetable stocks or broths as a base and loading the dish with a variety of colorful vegetables. This not only boosts the antioxidant content but also creates a visually appealing meal that is both satisfying and healthy, perfect for anyone aiming to maintain a balanced diabetic diet.

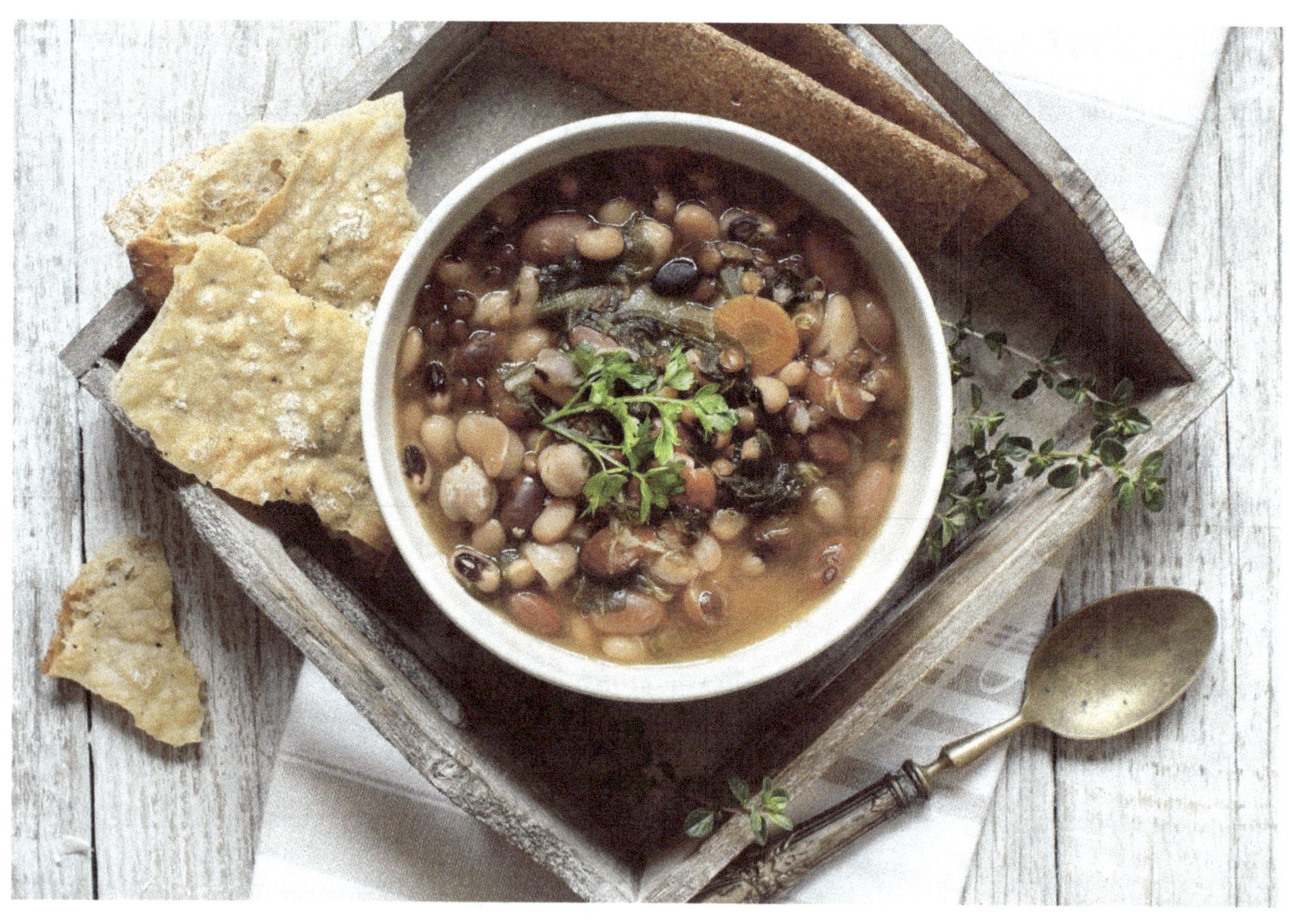

The Mediterranean diet, known for its heart-healthy benefits, also provides a wealth of inspiration for hearty soups and stews. Ingredients such as tomatoes, olive oil, garlic, and herbs are foundational to Mediterranean cooking and can easily be incorporated into various recipes. A Mediterranean-inspired vegetable and chickpea stew, for instance, can be both filling and nutritious, featuring a blend of spices that enhances flavor without adding excessive carbohydrates. This approach not only adheres to diabetic dietary guidelines but also introduces a variety of international flavors that can make meal preparation more enjoyable.

When planning meals, consider batch cooking soups and stews to support a successful diabetic meal prep strategy. Preparing large quantities allows for quick, convenient options throughout the week, reducing the temptation to reach for less healthy alternatives. Soups and stews can be portioned and frozen, making them an ideal choice for individuals practicing intermittent fasting or those looking to streamline their cooking efforts. Labeling containers with nutritional information can help in maintaining portion control and ensuring meals fit within diabetes-friendly guidelines.

Finally, it is essential to be mindful of ingredient choices when crafting hearty soups and stews. Opting for gluten-free grains, such as quinoa or brown rice, can offer additional texture and flavor without the adverse effects associated with gluten. Additionally, exploring culturally specific recipes can introduce new ingredients and cooking techniques that keep meals fresh and exciting. By prioritizing nutritious components and being thoughtful about preparation methods, hearty soups and stews can become a beloved part of any diabetic meal plan, providing nourishment and comfort in equal measure.

Easy Meat and Vegetable Dishes

Easy meat and vegetable dishes are an essential component of a diabetic-friendly diet, offering simplicity and versatility while emphasizing nutrient-dense ingredients. When preparing meals, it is crucial to focus on lean proteins and a variety of colorful vegetables, both of which provide essential vitamins and minerals. These dishes can help maintain stable blood sugar levels while ensuring that meals are satisfying and flavorful. By incorporating herbs and spices, one can elevate the taste without the need for excessive fats or sugars, making healthy eating both enjoyable and sustainable.

A foundational aspect of creating easy meat and vegetable dishes is selecting the right proteins. Lean meats such as chicken breast, turkey, and fish are excellent choices, providing necessary protein without the added saturated fats found in red meats. Plant-based proteins such as lentils, chickpeas, and tofu also serve as fantastic alternatives, especially within the Mediterranean diet framework. These options not only contribute to lower carbohydrate intake but also offer high fiber content, which is beneficial for digestion and blood sugar management.

Incorporating a variety of vegetables into your meals enhances both nutrition and flavor. Non-starchy vegetables such as spinach, broccoli, zucchini, and bell peppers are particularly beneficial for diabetics, as they are low in carbohydrates and high in fiber. Roasting or steaming vegetables can bring out their natural flavors, while a sprinkle of olive oil and a mix of herbs can create a delicious and healthy side dish. For those following plant-based or Mediterranean diets, creating hearty vegetable-based dishes such as ratatouille or stuffed peppers can satisfy both hunger and nutritional needs.

Meal prep strategies can significantly simplify the process of preparing easy meat and vegetable dishes. Setting aside time each week to wash, chop, and store vegetables can save time during busy weekdays. Cooking larger batches of proteins, such as grilled chicken or baked fish, allows for versatile meal options throughout the week. These prepped ingredients can be easily combined into salads, stir-fries, or wraps, ensuring that meals remain diverse and interesting without the stress of daily cooking.

Finally, incorporating healthy snacks into your diet can complement easy meat and vegetable dishes. Diabetic-friendly snack options such as hummus with carrot sticks or Greek yogurt with berries can help manage hunger between meals. These snacks are not only low in carbohydrates but also rich in protein and healthy fats, supporting overall health and energy levels. By focusing on easy, nutrient-rich meat and vegetable dishes, individuals can create a balanced and satisfying meal plan that aligns with their dietary needs and preferences, paving the way for better diabetes management.

Chapter 7:
The Mediterranean Diet and Diabetes

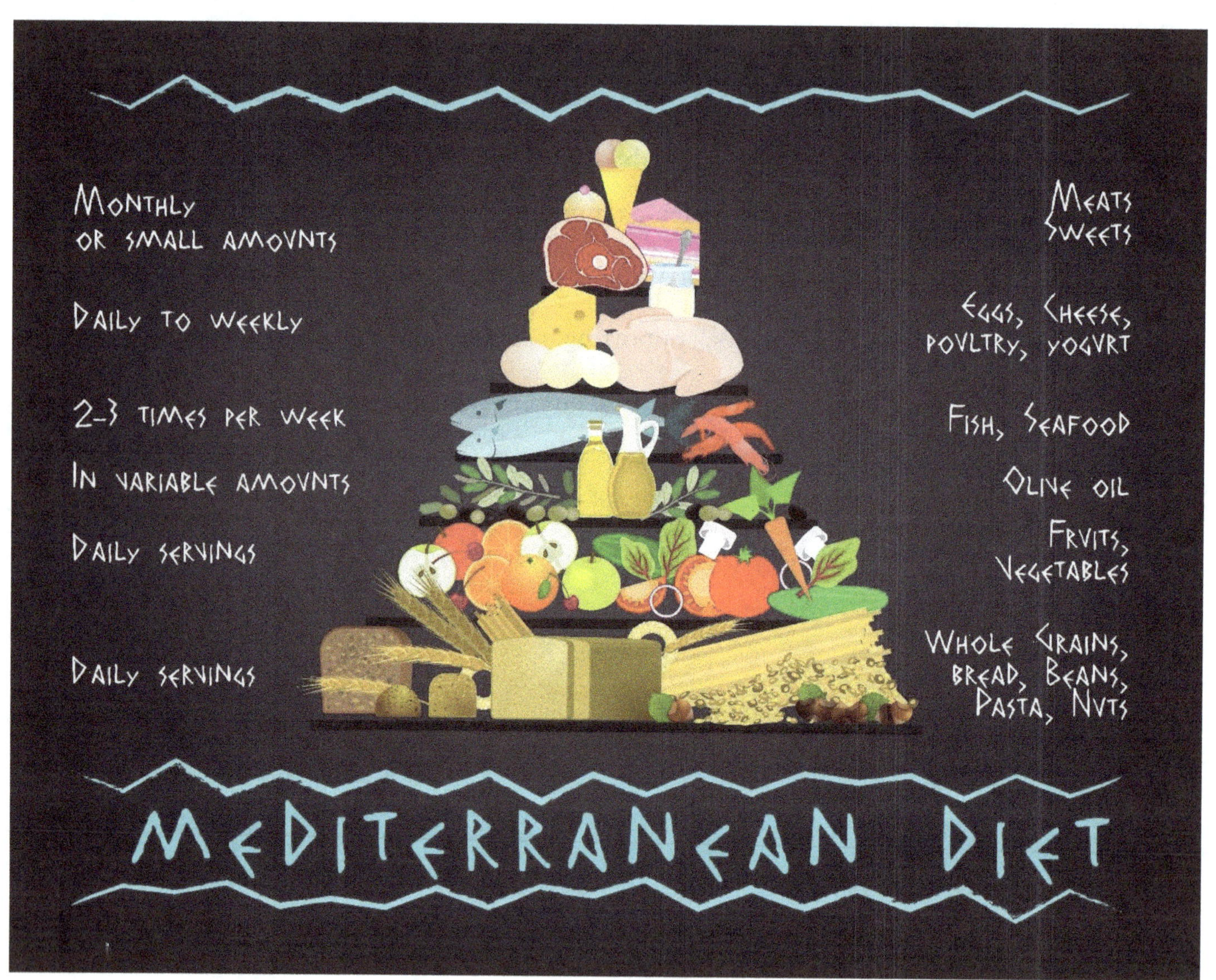

Principles of the Mediterranean Diet

The Mediterranean diet is not only a culinary delight but also a nutritional powerhouse that aligns well with diabetes management.

Characterized by an abundance of plant-based foods, healthy fats, and lean proteins, this diet emphasizes whole, unprocessed ingredients that can help regulate blood sugar levels. By focusing on fruits, vegetables, whole grains, legumes, nuts, and olive oil, individuals can enjoy meals that are rich in vitamins, minerals, and antioxidants. The principles of the Mediterranean diet promote a balanced approach to eating, making it a suitable option for those seeking to manage diabetes through dietary choices.

One of the core principles of the Mediterranean diet is the inclusion of healthy fats, particularly monounsaturated fats found in olive oil. These fats can improve insulin sensitivity and reduce inflammation, which is crucial for individuals with diabetes. Unlike saturated fats, which can raise cholesterol levels and increase the risk of heart disease, the fats in this diet contribute to overall cardiovascular health. Incorporating olive oil as a primary source of fat in cooking and dressings not only enhances flavor but also supports better glycemic control.

The Mediterranean diet also encourages the consumption of whole grains over refined carbohydrates. Whole grains such as quinoa, barley, and brown rice provide essential fiber, which aids in digestion and helps maintain steady blood sugar levels. By choosing these complex carbohydrates, individuals can experience a slower release of glucose into the bloodstream, reducing the risk of spikes in blood sugar. This focus on fiber-rich foods is particularly beneficial for those managing diabetes, as it promotes satiety and can assist in weight management.

Fruits and vegetables are the foundation of the Mediterranean diet, offering a wide array of nutrients while being naturally low in calories and carbohydrates. Non-starchy vegetables like spinach, kale, and bell peppers contribute to a vibrant, nutrient-dense plate that supports overall health. Fruits, particularly berries and citrus, provide antioxidants and can satisfy sweet cravings without causing significant blood sugar increases. The emphasis on seasonal and locally sourced produce encourages a diverse intake of nutrients, which is essential for optimal health in individuals with diabetes.

Finally, the Mediterranean diet promotes a lifestyle that encourages mindful eating and social interactions during meals. Sharing food with family and friends fosters a sense of community and enjoyment, which can enhance the overall eating experience. This principle aligns well with intermittent fasting practices, where meal timing and preparation can be thoughtfully planned to support diabetes management. By integrating these principles into daily life, individuals can create a sustainable and enjoyable eating plan that not only helps in managing diabetes but also enhances overall well-being.

Health Benefits for Diabetics

Health benefits for diabetics are multifaceted, encompassing physical, emotional, and social dimensions. A well-structured diet plays a critical role in managing blood glucose levels, reducing the risk of complications, and improving overall quality of life. By focusing on a diabetic-friendly meal plan, individuals can effectively control their weight, enhance their energy levels, and foster a sense of well-being. This subchapter will explore how various dietary approaches, including low-carb options, plant-based diets, and the Mediterranean diet, contribute to better health outcomes for those living with diabetes.

Low-carbohydrate meal plans are particularly beneficial for diabetics as they help stabilize blood sugar levels by minimizing insulin spikes. By reducing the intake of refined carbohydrates and sugars, individuals can better manage their glycemic response. Foods rich in fiber, such as non-starchy vegetables, legumes, and whole grains, provide essential nutrients while promoting satiety. Additionally, focusing on protein-rich foods aids in muscle maintenance and can support metabolic health, making low-carb diets an effective strategy for weight management and diabetes control.

Plant-based diets have gained recognition for their potential to improve diabetes management. These diets emphasize whole foods, including fruits, vegetables, nuts, seeds, and whole grains, which are inherently low in saturated fats and high in fiber. The antioxidants and phytochemicals found in plant-based foods can reduce inflammation and enhance insulin sensitivity. For many individuals with diabetes, adopting a plant-based approach not only aids in blood sugar control but also promotes cardiovascular health, making it a holistic choice for long-term wellness.

The Mediterranean diet, characterized by its emphasis on healthy fats, lean proteins, and a variety of fruits and vegetables, has also shown promise for diabetics. This dietary pattern supports heart health while helping to regulate blood sugar levels. Olive oil, nuts, and fatty fish provide essential omega-3 fatty acids, which can improve lipid profiles and reduce the risk of heart disease, a common concern for individuals with diabetes. Furthermore, the Mediterranean diet encourages social eating and cultural traditions, enhancing the overall dining experience and making healthy eating more enjoyable.

Lastly, incorporating diabetic-friendly snacks and desserts into a meal plan can satisfy cravings without compromising health. Options such as Greek yogurt with berries or almond butter on whole grain crackers offer balance and nutrition. Moreover, strategies like meal prepping and intermittent fasting can aid in maintaining consistency and controlling calorie intake. By embracing a variety of culturally specific recipes and nutritional supplements tailored for diabetics, individuals can create a sustainable and enjoyable dietary lifestyle that supports their health and well-being in managing diabetes effectively.

Mediterranean Meal Ideas

The Mediterranean diet is widely recognized for its health benefits, particularly for those managing diabetes. This diet emphasizes whole foods, healthy fats, and a variety of plant-based ingredients, making it an excellent choice for individuals looking to maintain stable blood sugar levels. When planning meals, consider incorporating an array of fresh vegetables, legumes, whole grains, and lean proteins. Staples such as olive oil, nuts, and seeds not only enhance flavors but also provide heart-healthy fats that are crucial for overall well-being.

For breakfast, a Mediterranean-inspired meal could include a vegetable omelet made with fresh spinach, tomatoes, and bell peppers, paired with a slice of whole-grain toast. This combination provides protein, fiber, and essential vitamins, setting a balanced tone for the day. Alternatively, consider a Greek yogurt parfait layered with berries and a sprinkle of chia seeds for added fiber and omega-3 fatty acids. This meal is not only satisfying but also supports digestive health, which is vital for maintaining stable glucose levels.

Lunch options can include a quinoa salad tossed with cucumbers, olives, red onion, and a drizzle of lemon-olive oil dressing. Quinoa is a great source of protein and fiber, which helps to regulate blood sugar levels. For those looking for something warm, a lentil soup made with diced tomatoes, carrots, and celery can be both filling and nutritious. Lentils are rich in protein and low on the glycemic index, making them an ideal choice for a diabetic-friendly meal.

Dinner could feature grilled chicken or fish marinated in herbs and lemon, served alongside a medley of roasted vegetables such as zucchini, eggplant, and bell peppers.

This meal not only provides lean protein but also allows for an abundance of vitamins and minerals. For a low-carb twist, consider substituting traditional pasta with spiralized zucchini or spaghetti squash, topped with a light tomato sauce and fresh basil. Such meals are not only diabetic-friendly but also align with Mediterranean dietary principles.

Snacking can also be approached with a Mediterranean flair. Options include hummus paired with raw vegetables or whole-grain pita chips, providing a nutritious and satisfying snack. Another choice is a handful of mixed nuts, which offer healthy fats and protein, helping to curb hunger between meals. For those with a sweet tooth, a small serving of dark chocolate or a fruit salad with a sprinkle of cinnamon can serve as a delicious and diabetes-friendly dessert. By integrating these Mediterranean meal ideas into your daily routine, you can enjoy flavorful dishes that support your diabetic management goals.

Chapter 8:
Diabetic-Friendly Snack Options

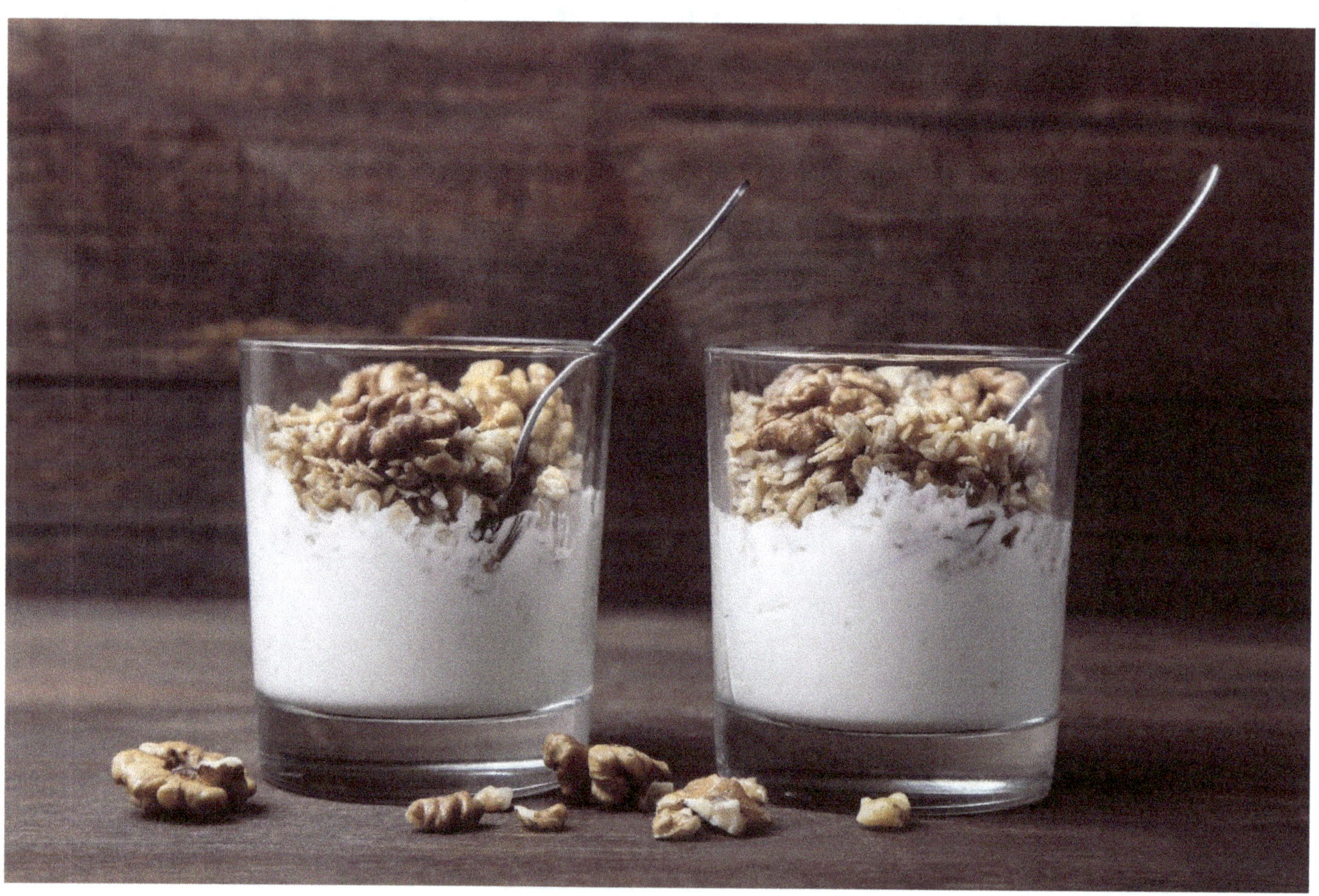

Importance of Healthy Snacking

Healthy snacking plays a crucial role in managing diabetes and can significantly impact overall health and well-being. For individuals navigating the complexities of a diabetic diet, choosing the right snacks can help maintain stable blood sugar levels, prevent overeating during meals, and provide essential nutrients.

This is particularly important for both men and women who may have different nutritional needs and lifestyle considerations. By incorporating healthy snacks into their daily routines, individuals can better control their hunger and energy levels, making it easier to adhere to their meal plans.

When selecting snacks, it is vital to focus on low-carb options that align with diabetic dietary guidelines. Snacks that are rich in protein, fiber, and healthy fats can help slow the absorption of carbohydrates, leading to more stable blood sugar readings. Options such as nuts, seeds, Greek yogurt, and raw vegetables are excellent choices that can be easily integrated into any meal plan. These snacks not only provide essential nutrients but also contribute to satiety, which can be particularly beneficial for those practicing intermittent fasting or following specific meal prep strategies.

Plant-based diets have gained popularity among those managing diabetes, and healthy snacking can seamlessly fit into this approach. Incorporating fruits, vegetables, and whole grains into snacks can provide valuable vitamins and minerals while remaining low in refined sugars and unhealthy fats. Additionally, Mediterranean-inspired snacks, such as hummus with vegetable sticks or whole grain crackers with olive oil, offer flavorful and nutritious options that support heart health and diabetes management. These snacks can enhance dietary variety while encouraging a balanced, healthful eating pattern.

Culturally specific diabetic diets can also inform healthy snacking choices. Many traditional cuisines offer nutrient-dense options that can be adapted to meet diabetic needs. For example, incorporating legumes, whole grains, and fresh herbs into snack choices can provide an authentic taste while promoting health. By embracing these cultural foods, individuals can enjoy their heritage while adhering to dietary restrictions, making healthy snacking an enjoyable part of their journey.

Lastly, it is essential to consider the role of nutritional supplements in complementing healthy snacking habits. For those with specific dietary restrictions or challenges in meeting their nutritional needs, supplements can provide an additional layer of support. Ensuring that snacks are balanced with the right nutrients can help in managing blood sugar levels and overall health. By prioritizing healthy snacking, individuals can create a more sustainable and enjoyable approach to their diabetic meal plans, paving the way for long-term success in diabetes management.

Quick and Easy Snack Recipes

Quick and easy snacks are essential for maintaining stable blood sugar levels while satisfying cravings. For individuals managing diabetes, choosing snacks that align with dietary goals can be challenging. The focus should be on low-carb, nutrient-dense options that provide energy without causing significant spikes in blood sugar. This subchapter presents a selection of quick and easy snack recipes that cater to various dietary preferences, including plant-based and Mediterranean diets, while ensuring they remain diabetic-friendly.

One simple yet satisfying option is a cucumber and hummus snack. Slice fresh cucumbers and serve them with a portion of homemade or store-bought hummus. This combination offers a refreshing crunch along with a source of healthy fats and protein from the chickpeas in the hummus. This snack is not only low in carbohydrates but also rich in fiber, helping to promote satiety and stabilize blood sugar levels. For those following a gluten-free diet, ensure that the hummus is free from gluten-containing additives.

Another excellent quick snack is a handful of mixed nuts. Nuts are a great source of healthy fats, protein, and fiber, making them a perfect choice for those on a low-carb diabetic meal plan. A mixture of almonds, walnuts, and pistachios can provide a variety of nutrients, including magnesium, which has been shown to support insulin sensitivity. It is important to keep portion sizes in check, as nuts are calorie-dense, but a small serving can curb hunger and provide sustained energy.

For a sweet yet diabetic-friendly treat, consider Greek yogurt topped with berries. Opt for plain, unsweetened yogurt to avoid added sugars, and add a small handful of fresh or frozen berries. Berries are lower in carbohydrates compared to other fruits and are packed with antioxidants, making them a smart choice for a snack. This combination also provides protein from the yogurt, promoting fullness and helping to maintain stable blood sugar levels. Those following a Mediterranean diet will particularly appreciate this nutritious option.

Finally, a quick and easy snack can be made by preparing avocado toast on gluten-free bread. Mash half an avocado and spread it on a slice of gluten-free bread or a rice cake, and top it with a sprinkle of salt, pepper, and optional seeds, such as chia or flaxseed. This snack is rich in healthy fats and fiber, promoting heart health and aiding in blood sugar control. Avocados are also known for their low glycemic index, making them suitable for individuals needing to manage their carbohydrate intake.

These quick and easy snack recipes not only align with diabetic dietary requirements but also cater to a variety of preferences and lifestyle choices. Incorporating these snacks into daily routines can lead to better blood sugar management while offering enjoyable and flavorful options. As with any dietary changes, monitoring individual responses and adjusting portion sizes as needed is key to success in diabetes management.

Smart Snacking Strategies

Smart snacking is an essential component of managing diabetes effectively while still enjoying the foods you love. For both men and women navigating a diabetic diet, understanding how to select snacks wisely can make a significant difference in blood sugar levels and overall health. The key is to focus on nutrient-dense options that are low in carbohydrates, high in fiber, and packed with healthy fats and proteins. This not only promotes satiety but also helps stabilize blood sugar levels throughout the day.

Incorporating a variety of diabetic-friendly snacks into your meal plan can prevent the temptation of reaching for less nutritious options. Think of snacks as opportunities to boost your intake of vitamins, minerals, and antioxidants. For instance, consider raw vegetables paired with hummus or a small handful of nuts. These snacks are not only low in carbohydrates but also provide essential nutrients and healthy fats that can help control hunger without causing spikes in blood sugar levels.

Plant-based snacks can be particularly beneficial for those following a diabetic diet. Foods such as edamame, chickpeas, or a small serving of guacamole with vegetables can deliver a satisfying crunch while promoting heart health.

For individuals considering gluten-free options, there are numerous snacks that cater to both dietary restrictions and the need for blood sugar control. Rice cakes topped with almond butter or a small bowl of quinoa salad with vegetables can keep you nourished without compromising your health goals. Furthermore, for those interested in intermittent fasting, planning your snacks around your eating windows can help ensure that you are consuming balanced, diabetic-friendly options that provide sustained energy.

Finally, preparation is key in fostering smart snacking habits. Meal prepping snacks ahead of time can eliminate the last-minute scramble for food choices that might not align with your dietary needs. Designate a day each week to prepare snacks like veggie portions or portion-controlled fruit servings. By having ready-to-eat, diabetes-friendly snacks on hand, you can maintain better control over your dietary choices and ensure that you are fueling your body with the right nutrients at the right times.

Chapter 9:
Gluten-Free Diabetic Recipes

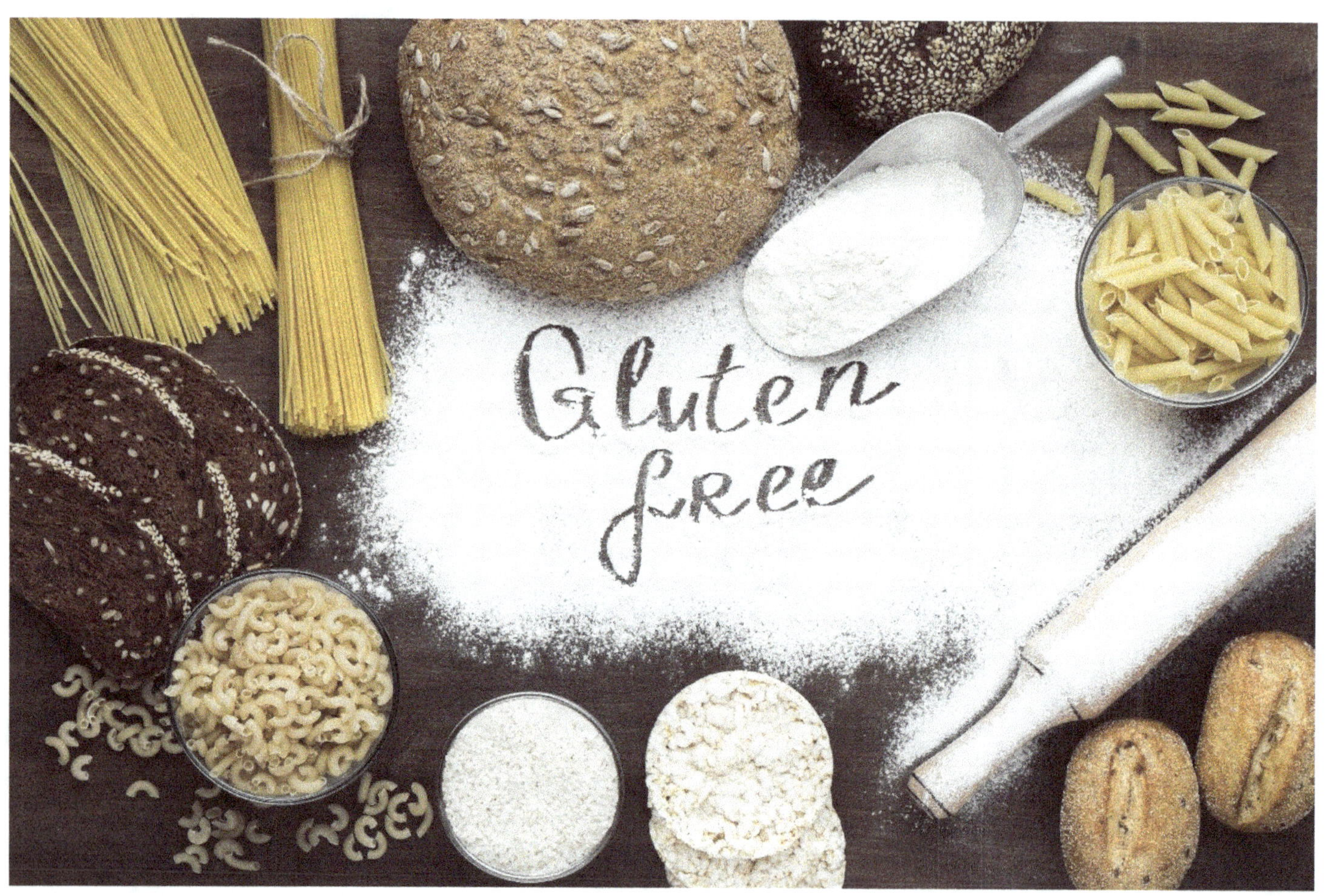

Gluten-Free Meal Ideas

Incorporating gluten-free meal ideas into a diabetic diet can enhance nutritional quality while accommodating specific dietary needs. Individuals managing diabetes often seek meals that stabilize blood sugar levels without sacrificing taste or variety.

Gluten-free options can include an array of whole foods that align with diabetic-friendly guidelines, promoting overall health. By focusing on low-carb ingredients and nutrient-dense choices, it becomes easier to craft meals that are both satisfying and beneficial.

A foundational aspect of gluten-free meal preparation is the use of whole grains and legumes that naturally lack gluten. Quinoa, brown rice, and lentils are excellent bases for salads or grain bowls, providing essential fiber and protein. For a Mediterranean twist, consider a quinoa tabbouleh salad with cucumbers, tomatoes, and fresh herbs, dressed with olive oil and lemon juice. This dish not only meets gluten-free requirements but also aligns with low-carb and plant-based principles, making it an ideal choice for those looking to manage their diabetes effectively.

In addition to main dishes, snack options play a crucial role in a diabetic meal plan. Gluten-free snacks can be both nutritious and satisfying. Hummus served with sliced veggies or gluten-free crackers is a perfect choice, offering healthy fats and protein to curb hunger. Another option is Greek yogurt topped with berries and a sprinkle of cinnamon, which provides a low-sugar alternative that satisfies sweet cravings without compromising blood sugar control. These snacks can be easily prepared in advance, supporting meal prep strategies that save time and ensure healthy choices are always on hand.

For those interested in cultural cuisines, many traditional dishes easily adapt to gluten-free and diabetic-friendly options. For instance, Mexican cuisine offers a variety of naturally gluten-free ingredients, such as corn tortillas, beans, and fresh vegetables. A black bean and corn salad, spiced with lime and cilantro, serves as a flavorful side dish or a light main course. Similarly, Asian cuisines can provide gluten-free alternatives by utilizing rice noodles or vegetable stir-fries, ensuring that meals remain diverse and enjoyable while adhering to dietary restrictions.

Desserts do not have to be neglected in a gluten-free diabetic meal plan. A simple yet delightful option could be almond flour cookies sweetened with a sugar substitute.

These treats maintain flavor while being mindful of carbohydrate content. Additionally, fruit-based desserts, such as a berry compote served over a dollop of Greek yogurt, can satisfy the sweet tooth without the drawbacks of traditional sugary desserts. By integrating these gluten-free meal ideas, individuals can foster a balanced approach to their diabetic diet, enhancing their overall health and enjoyment of food.

Baking and Cooking Without Gluten

Baking and cooking without gluten presents a unique opportunity to create delicious and nutritious meals that cater to diabetic dietary needs. Gluten, found in wheat, barley, and rye, can be challenging for individuals who also need to manage their blood sugar levels. By focusing on gluten-free ingredients, one can explore a variety of alternative flours such as almond, coconut, and chickpea flour, which not only provide a gluten-free option but also contribute to a lower carbohydrate content. Incorporating these flours into your baking and cooking can help maintain stable blood sugar levels while still enjoying flavorful dishes.

When baking, it is essential to understand the functional differences between gluten-free flours and traditional flours. Gluten provides elasticity and structure, which can be challenging to replicate. Therefore, using a combination of gluten-free flours, along with binding agents like xanthan gum or psyllium husk, can help achieve the desired texture in baked goods. Additionally, experimenting with moisture levels and cooking times may be necessary to perfect recipes.

This adjustment process can lead to the discovery of new favorite dishes that align with a diabetic-friendly diet.

In the realm of savory cooking, gluten-free grains and legumes can serve as excellent substitutes for traditional pasta and bread. Options such as quinoa, brown rice, and lentils not only offer a gluten-free alternative but also enhance the nutritional profile of meals. These ingredients are rich in fiber, which is beneficial for blood sugar control and can help you feel fuller for longer. Pairing these grains with plenty of vegetables and healthy fats, common in the Mediterranean diet, results in satisfying meals that support overall health and well-being.

Snacking is another area where gluten-free options can shine. Many traditional snacks contain gluten and are high in carbohydrates, which can lead to blood sugar spikes. However, by preparing diabetic-friendly snacks such as roasted chickpeas, vegetable sticks with hummus, or gluten-free energy bites made from nuts and seeds, individuals can enjoy satisfying treats without compromising their health. These snacks can be easily incorporated into meal prep strategies, making them convenient for busy lifestyles while ensuring that they align with dietary goals.

Finally, desserts should not be overlooked in a gluten-free and diabetic-friendly approach. By utilizing naturally sweet ingredients such as ripe bananas, applesauce, or dark chocolate, one can create decadent treats without the need for gluten or excessive sugar. Recipes for gluten-free brownies, chia seed puddings, and coconut flour cookies can delight the palate while still being mindful of carbohydrate intake. With careful ingredient selection and thoughtful preparation, it is entirely possible to enjoy a wide array of baked goods and meals that are both gluten-free and suitable for managing diabetes.

Chapter 10:
Vegan and Vegetarian Diabetic Diet Recipes

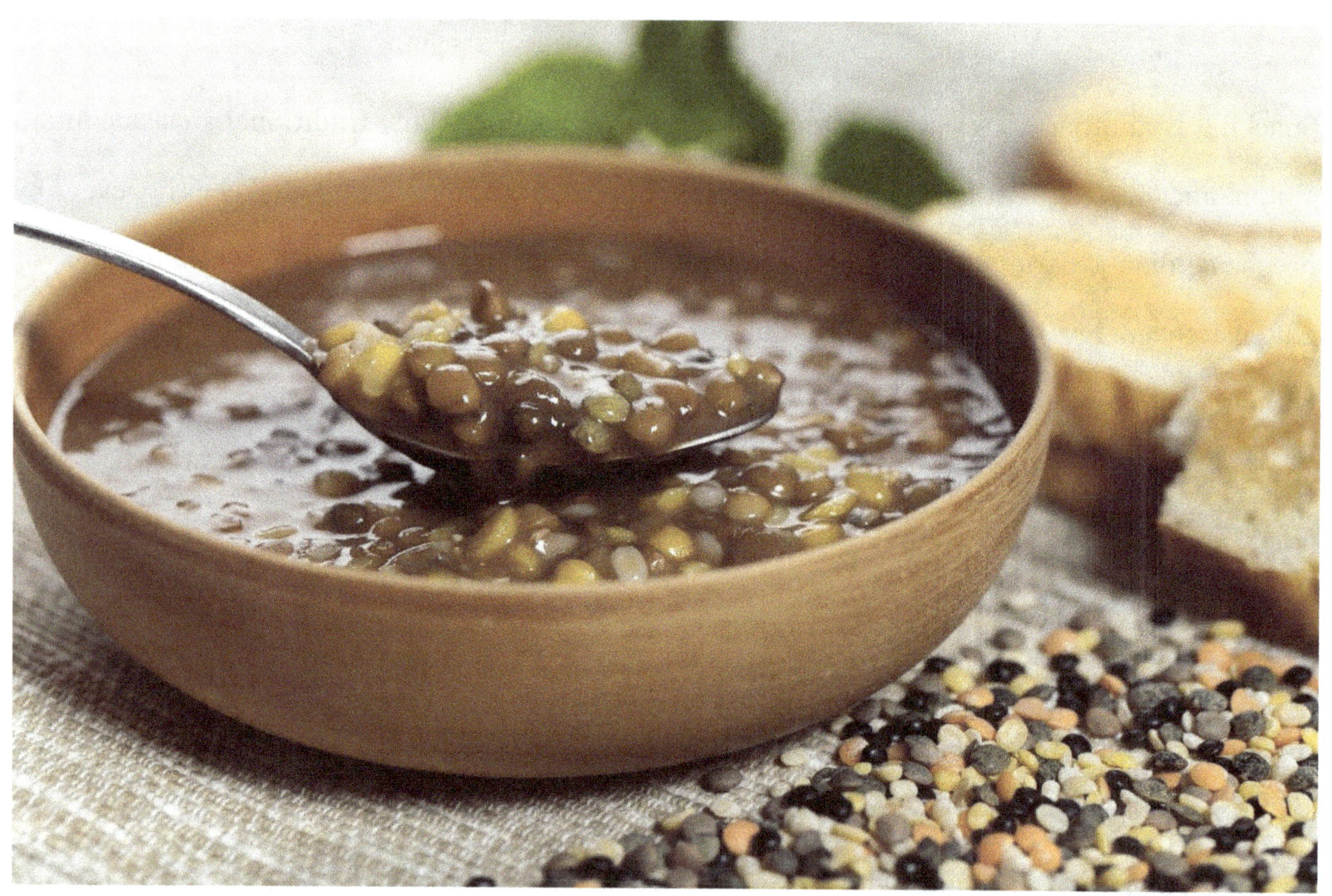

Plant-Based Breakfasts

Plant-based breakfasts can be an excellent choice for individuals managing diabetes, as they are typically low in carbohydrates and rich in nutrients. Incorporating a variety of whole foods such as fruits, vegetables, whole grains, nuts, and seeds can help stabilize blood sugar levels and provide sustained energy throughout the day.

A well-planned plant-based breakfast not only supports diabetes management but also aligns with a Mediterranean-inspired diet, which emphasizes healthy fats, fiber, and a plethora of vitamins and minerals.

One popular plant-based breakfast option is overnight oats. By combining rolled oats with unsweetened almond milk, chia seeds, and a selection of berries, individuals can create a hearty meal that is low in sugar and high in fiber. The fiber content helps to slow down the absorption of carbohydrates, preventing sharp spikes in blood glucose levels. This dish can be prepared in advance, making it ideal for those practicing meal prep strategies and looking to save time during busy mornings.

Another nutritious option includes a vegetable-packed tofu scramble. By sautéing a mix of spinach, bell peppers, and onions with firm tofu, individuals can enjoy a savory breakfast that is both satisfying and protein-rich. Tofu is an excellent source of plant-based protein and contains minimal carbohydrates, making it suitable for those following low-carb diabetic meal plans. Additionally, spices such as turmeric and black pepper not only enhance flavor but also offer anti-inflammatory benefits, which can be advantageous for overall health.

Smoothies provide a versatile and quick breakfast choice for busy mornings. A combination of leafy greens, such as kale or spinach, blended with unsweetened plant-based yogurt, a small serving of nuts, and a low-glycemic fruit like berries can create a refreshing start to the day. This nutrient-dense beverage can be easily customized according to personal preferences, making it possible to include various nutrient-dense ingredients such as flaxseeds or hemp seeds, further enhancing its health benefits for diabetes management.

For those seeking sweet options, chia seed pudding can serve as a delightful and diabetes-friendly dessert for breakfast. By mixing chia seeds with unsweetened almond milk and a touch of vanilla extract, this dish can be left to thicken overnight. Topped with a handful of nuts or a sprinkle of cinnamon, chia seed pudding offers a delightful balance of healthy fats, fiber, and protein, making it an ideal choice for maintaining stable blood sugar levels. By exploring these plant-based breakfast ideas, individuals can enjoy delicious and nutritious meals while effectively managing their diabetes.

Wholesome Lunches

Wholesome lunches play a crucial role in managing diabetes, offering not only essential nutrients but also the satisfaction needed to prevent mid-afternoon energy slumps. Crafting a lunch that aligns with diabetic dietary needs involves careful selection of ingredients that promote stable blood sugar levels while providing a variety of flavors and textures. Emphasizing low-carb options, plant-based ingredients, and Mediterranean influences can make lunchtime both enjoyable and nourishing.

A well-balanced diabetic-friendly lunch should incorporate lean proteins, healthy fats, and plenty of non-starchy vegetables. For example, a quinoa salad topped with grilled chicken, feta cheese, and a medley of colorful vegetables can serve as a filling yet low-carb option. The inclusion of olive oil and lemon juice not only enhances the flavors but also contributes to heart health, aligning with Mediterranean dietary principles. Such meals can keep blood sugar levels stable while providing sustained energy throughout the day.

Incorporating whole foods into lunch preparation is essential for anyone following a diabetic diet. Whole grains, such as farro or brown rice, can be combined with legumes like chickpeas or lentils to create hearty bowls that are both satisfying and nutritious. These ingredients are excellent sources of fiber, which aids in digestion and helps control blood sugar spikes. Moreover, seasoning with herbs and spices instead of relying on salt enhances the meal's flavor without compromising health.

For those interested in meal prep strategies, creating large batches of wholesome lunches can save time during the week while ensuring that healthy options are readily available. Preparing components separately, such as proteins, grains, and vegetables, allows for customization and variety.

In addition, storing meals in portion-controlled containers can help manage serving sizes effectively, which is vital for blood sugar control. Including diabetic-friendly snacks, such as hummus with vegetable sticks or a handful of nuts, can complement lunches perfectly and keep hunger at bay.

Lastly, embracing cultural diversity in lunch preparation can enrich the diabetic diet experience. Exploring recipes from various cuisines, such as a Mediterranean-inspired wrap filled with roasted vegetables and tahini, or a spicy lentil soup from South Asian traditions, can introduce new flavors while adhering to dietary restrictions.

This approach not only makes meals more enjoyable but also encourages a broader understanding of nutrition and its role in diabetes management. By focusing on wholesome ingredients and diverse recipes, individuals can create lunches that are both satisfying and supportive of their health goals.

Satisfying Dinners

Satisfying dinners are an essential component of a diabetic diet, offering not only nutritional balance but also the joy of a fulfilling meal. For individuals managing diabetes, it is crucial to focus on meals that are low in carbohydrates while also being rich in flavor and variety.

Incorporating vegetables, lean proteins, and healthy fats can help regulate blood sugar levels, ensuring that dinner is both enjoyable and healthy. By prioritizing whole foods and minimizing processed options, individuals can craft dinners that not only satisfy hunger but also support overall health.

A low-carb diabetic meal plan can effectively manage blood sugar levels while providing a diverse array of flavors and textures. Dinner recipes may include grilled chicken or fish served alongside a vibrant array of roasted non-starchy vegetables. For those who enjoy plant-based diets, legumes and whole grains can serve as excellent protein sources. Quinoa, lentils, and chickpeas are not only high in fiber but also help in maintaining satiety. Additionally, incorporating herbs and spices can enhance the flavors of these dishes, making even simple meals extraordinary.

The Mediterranean diet, known for its heart-healthy benefits, is particularly suitable for diabetics. This approach emphasizes the consumption of olive oil, whole grains, fish, and an abundance of fruits and vegetables. A satisfying dinner could feature a Mediterranean grain bowl filled with farro, roasted vegetables, and a drizzle of tahini or yogurt dressing. Such meals are not only delicious but also provide essential nutrients that contribute to better glycemic control. Furthermore, the use of portion control and mindful eating practices can enhance the dining experience, allowing individuals to appreciate their meals fully.

For those looking to prepare meals in advance, meal prep strategies can be a game-changer in maintaining a diabetic-friendly diet. Preparing larger batches of meals can save time and ensure that healthy options are readily available during busy weekdays. Dinners can be portioned out into containers, allowing for quick reheating while still being nutritious. Including a variety of flavors and ingredients in these prepped meals helps to combat monotony, making it easier to stick with a healthy eating plan.

Desserts can also play a role in satisfying dinner experiences. Diabetic-friendly dessert options, such as fruit-based treats or recipes using natural sweeteners like stevia, can allow individuals to indulge without compromising their health. When planning satisfying dinners, it is essential to remember that balance is key. By including a nourishing main course, a colorful side dish, and a small dessert, individuals can create a fulfilling dining experience that supports their health goals while still enjoying the pleasures of food.

Chapter 11:

Intermittent Fasting for Diabetes Control

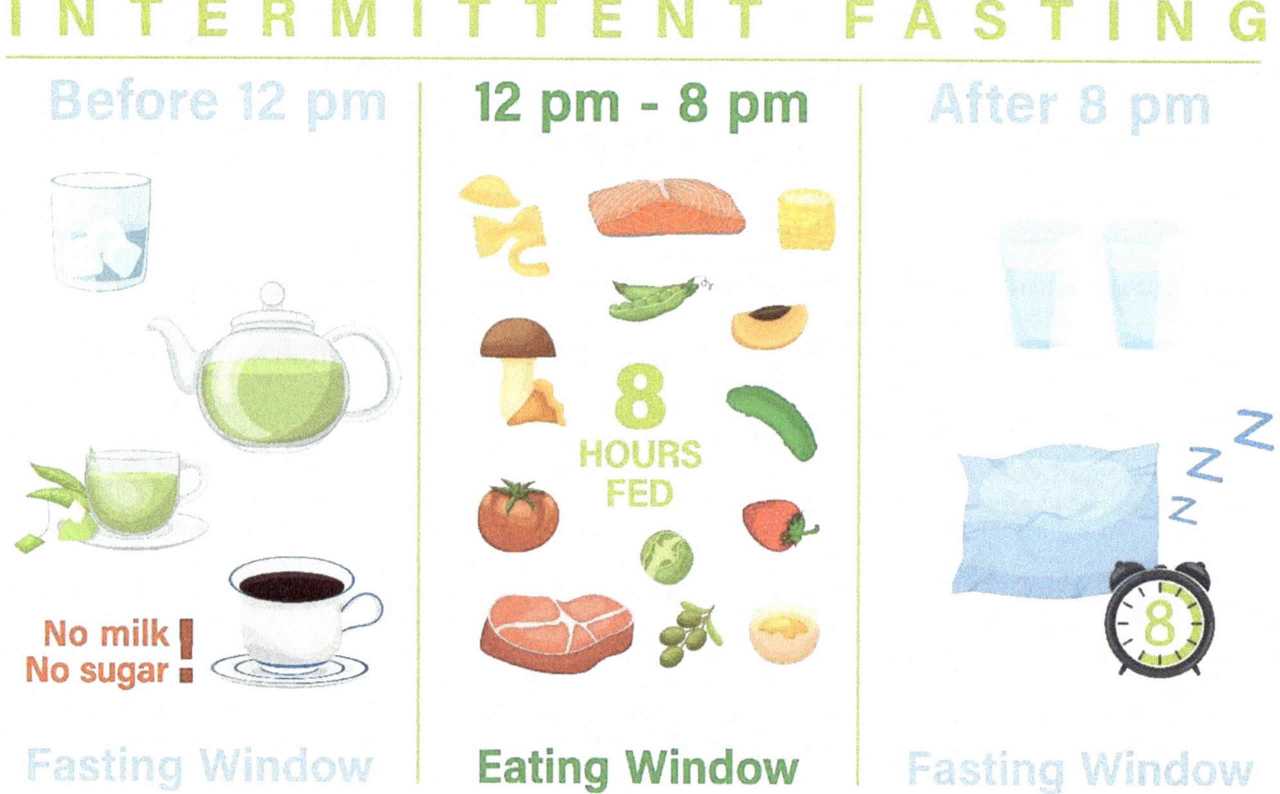

The Science Behind Intermittent Fasting

Intermittent fasting (IF) has gained significant attention in recent years as a viable strategy for managing various health conditions, including diabetes. The core principle of intermittent fasting involves cycling between periods of eating and fasting, which can promote various metabolic processes beneficial for blood sugar control.

For individuals with diabetes, understanding the science behind this approach is crucial for effectively incorporating it into their dietary plans. Research indicates that intermittent fasting may improve insulin sensitivity, decrease inflammation, and support weight management, all of which are critical factors in diabetes management.

During fasting periods, the body undergoes several physiological changes that can enhance metabolic health. When food intake is limited, insulin levels drop, facilitating fat breakdown and improving the body's ability to utilize stored energy. This process is particularly advantageous for individuals managing diabetes, as it can lead to more stable blood sugar levels. Additionally, intermittent fasting may initiate autophagy, a cellular repair process that helps remove damaged cells and regenerate new ones, potentially reducing the risk of diabetes-related complications.

In terms of dietary patterns, intermittent fasting can be seamlessly integrated with various dietary approaches suitable for individuals with diabetes. Whether one adheres to a low-carb meal plan, a plant-based diet, or a Mediterranean diet, intermittent fasting can complement these eating styles. For example, individuals following a Mediterranean diet can focus on nutrient-dense foods during their eating windows, such as fruits, vegetables, whole grains, and healthy fats, thereby enhancing the health benefits of both the diet and fasting. This combination can lead to improved glycemic control and overall well-being.

Moreover, the flexibility of intermittent fasting allows for personalization according to individual preferences and lifestyles. Different fasting schedules, such as the 16:8 method or alternate-day fasting, can cater to varying needs and help individuals maintain adherence. This adaptability is particularly important for those managing diabetes, as it enables them to choose a plan that aligns with their daily routines and food choices. By incorporating fasting into their lifestyles, individuals may find an effective method to enhance their diabetes management strategies without feeling deprived.

Finally, it is essential to approach intermittent fasting with careful consideration of one's overall dietary and health goals. While intermittent fasting holds promise for improving metabolic health in individuals with diabetes, it is not a one-size-fits-all solution. Consulting with healthcare providers and nutritionists can help tailor an intermittent fasting plan that aligns with dietary preferences and medical needs. By understanding the science behind intermittent fasting, individuals can make informed decisions that support their health and well-being, ultimately leading to improved diabetes management and quality of life.

Different Intermittent Fasting Methods

Intermittent fasting (IF) has gained popularity as a flexible eating pattern that can be particularly beneficial for people managing diabetes. Various methods of intermittent fasting allow individuals to choose an approach that best fits their lifestyles and preferences. Understanding these different methods is essential for effectively incorporating intermittent fasting into a diabetic meal plan. This subchapter will explore several popular intermittent fasting techniques, highlighting their unique characteristics and potential benefits for blood sugar management.

One widely practiced method is the 16/8 approach, where individuals fast for 16 hours each day and restrict their eating to an 8-hour window. For many, this means skipping breakfast and consuming meals between noon and 8 PM. This method can help stabilize insulin levels and reduce overall calorie intake, making it easier to maintain a healthy weight. By concentrating meals within a set time frame, individuals can also simplify meal planning, allowing for the selection of low-carb, diabetic-friendly options that align with their dietary needs.

Another common form is the 5:2 diet, which involves eating normally for five days of the week while restricting caloric intake to about 500-600 calories on two non-consecutive days. This method can be particularly appealing as it does not require daily fasting, making it easier for some to adhere to over the long term. On low-calorie days, individuals can focus on plant-based meals rich in fiber and nutrients, which can help manage hunger and maintain balanced blood sugar levels. This flexibility allows for the incorporation of diabetes-friendly snacks that are satisfying yet low in carbohydrates.

Alternate-day fasting is another approach where individuals alternate between fasting days and eating days. On fasting days, calorie intake is significantly reduced, while normal eating resumes the following day.

This method may be more challenging due to the drastic changes in eating patterns, but it can lead to substantial weight loss and improved insulin sensitivity over time. For those following a Mediterranean diet, incorporating healthy fats, lean proteins, and whole grains on eating days can further enhance the benefits of alternate-day fasting while providing essential nutrients.

The warrior diet offers a unique twist, where individuals fast for 20 hours and consume a large meal within a 4-hour window in the evening. This method is often associated with a more primal approach to eating, emphasizing whole, unprocessed foods and mindful consumption. For diabetics, focusing on nutrient-dense foods during the eating window is crucial to avoid spikes in blood sugar levels. This method encourages individuals to experiment with various recipes, including gluten-free options and diabetes-friendly desserts that can be enjoyed during the meal period.

In conclusion, different intermittent fasting methods provide various options for individuals looking to manage diabetes effectively. Each approach has its unique benefits and potential challenges, allowing for personalization based on individual preferences and lifestyle. By understanding these methods, individuals can integrate intermittent fasting into their dietary routines, promoting better blood sugar control while enjoying a variety of healthy, delicious meals that align with their nutritional goals.

Tips for Successful Fasting

Successful fasting can be a powerful tool for managing diabetes, but it requires careful planning and consideration to ensure safety and effectiveness. Individuals embarking on a fasting regimen should first consult with healthcare professionals to tailor their approach to their specific health needs. This step is critical to avoid potential complications, especially in those who are on medications or have other underlying health conditions. A well-thought-out fasting schedule can help stabilize blood sugar levels while allowing the body to adapt gradually to changes in meal timing.

When implementing fasting, it is essential to choose a method that fits one's lifestyle and dietary preferences. Intermittent fasting, for example, can be structured in various ways, such as the 16/8 method, where individuals fast for 16 hours and eat during an 8-hour window. This flexibility allows for the integration of low-carb or plant-based meals that align with diabetic dietary guidelines. Preparing meals in advance can aid in maintaining control over food choices during eating periods, ensuring that meals remain nutritious and compliant with diabetic requirements.

Hydration plays a pivotal role during fasting. It is crucial to consume adequate amounts of water, as dehydration can lead to fatigue and may impact blood sugar levels. Herbal teas or infusions can also be beneficial, providing both hydration and potential health benefits without added sugars. Additionally, incorporating low-calorie electrolytes can help maintain electrolyte balance during extended fasting periods, making the experience more comfortable and sustainable.

Monitoring blood sugar levels during fasting is vital for individuals with diabetes. Keeping a close eye on glucose readings can help identify how fasting impacts personal blood sugar management. It is advisable to have a plan in place for breaking the fast, ideally starting with a small, balanced meal that includes healthy fats, proteins, and low glycemic carbohydrates. This approach can help prevent spikes in blood sugar levels, ensuring that the transition back to regular eating is smooth and controlled.

Lastly, it is essential to listen to one's body throughout the fasting process. If feelings of dizziness, extreme hunger, or fatigue occur, it may be necessary to adjust the fasting schedule or seek guidance from a healthcare provider. Successful fasting for diabetes management is not just about following a regimen but also about understanding personal limits and making informed adjustments as needed. By embracing these tips, individuals can create a sustainable and effective fasting practice that supports their overall health and diabetes management goals.

Chapter 12:
Diabetic Meal Prep Strategies

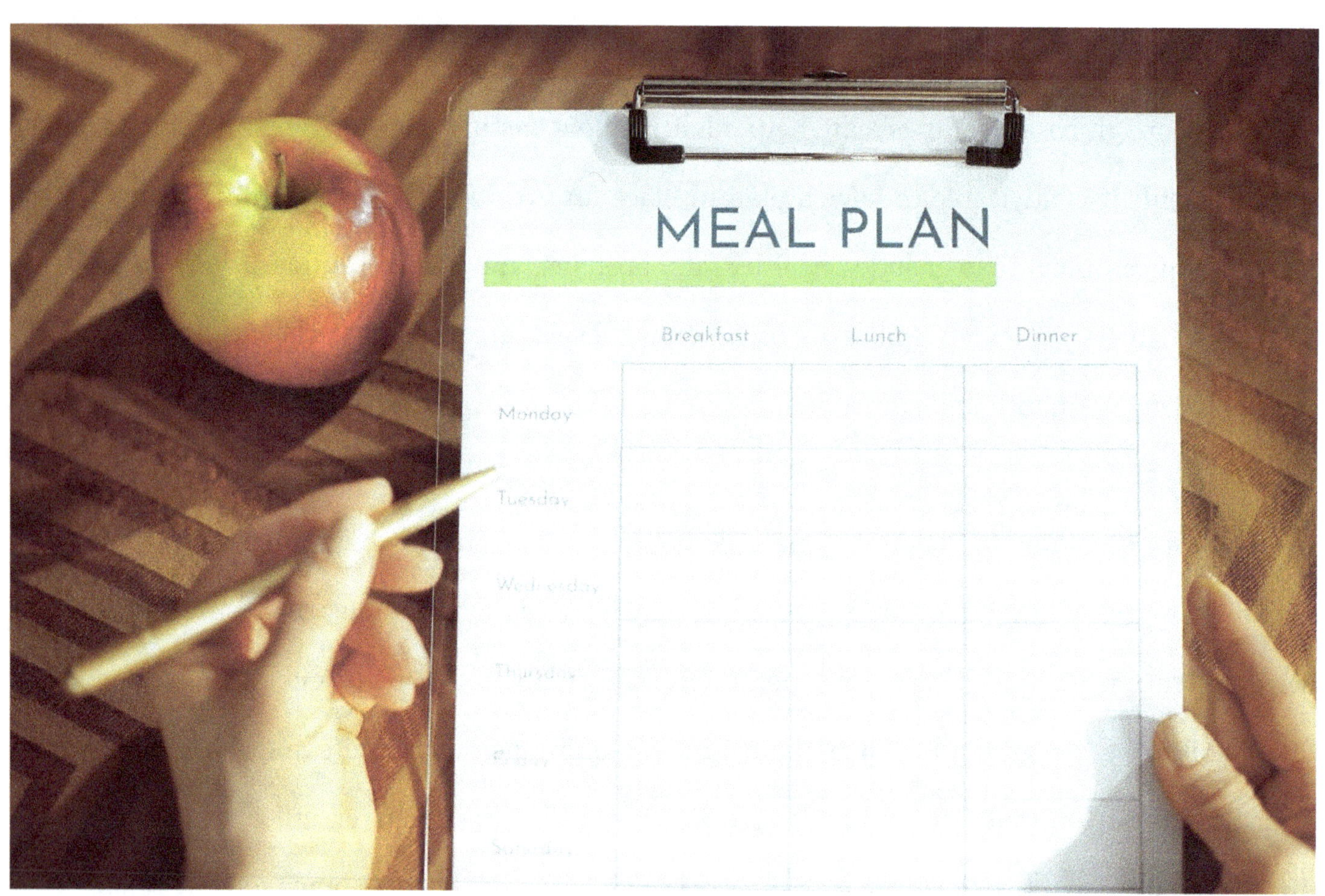

Benefits of Meal Prepping

Meal prepping offers numerous advantages for individuals managing diabetes, making it an essential strategy for maintaining a healthy lifestyle. One of the primary benefits is the control it provides over food choices and portion sizes.

By planning and preparing meals in advance, individuals can select ingredients that align with their dietary needs, ensuring adherence to low-carb, plant-based, or Mediterranean diets. This premeditated approach allows for better management of blood sugar levels, as meals can be tailored to include the right balance of carbohydrates, proteins, and healthy fats.

In addition to promoting better food choices, meal prepping significantly reduces the likelihood of impulsive eating and unhealthy snacking. When meals are prepared ahead of time, there is less temptation to reach for processed snacks or high-sugar foods. This is particularly beneficial for those on a diabetic diet, as it helps maintain stable blood sugar levels throughout the day. Moreover, having a variety of diabetic-friendly snacks ready to go can support adherence to dietary goals and provide satisfying options when hunger strikes.

Time management is another significant advantage of meal prepping. By dedicating a few hours each week to prepare meals, individuals can save time during busy weekdays. This efficiency not only simplifies daily routines but also alleviates the stress of last-minute cooking decisions, which can often lead to less healthy choices. With meals already prepared, individuals can focus on other important aspects of their lives, knowing that their nutritional needs are being met. Cost-effectiveness is also a noteworthy benefit of meal prepping. By planning meals and shopping for ingredients in advance, individuals can avoid the pitfalls of impulse purchases and reduce food waste. Buying ingredients in bulk and using seasonal produce can lead to significant savings, making it easier to maintain a budget while adhering to diabetes-friendly diets. Furthermore, preparing meals at home allows for greater control over ingredient quality and portion sizes, enhancing both health and financial well-being.

Finally, meal prepping fosters creativity and enjoyment in cooking, encouraging individuals to explore a variety of flavors and cuisines. Whether adapting culturally specific diabetic diets or experimenting with gluten-free recipes, meal prepping provides an opportunity to try new ingredients and dishes. This exploration can lead to discovering delicious diabetic-friendly desserts and snacks that satisfy cravings without compromising health. Ultimately, the benefits of meal prepping extend beyond mere convenience; they empower individuals to take charge of their health and make informed dietary choices that support their diabetes management journey.

Planning Your Weekly Meals

Planning your weekly meals is a crucial step in managing diabetes effectively. A well-structured meal plan not only helps maintain optimal blood sugar levels but also ensures a balanced intake of essential nutrients. Begin by evaluating your nutritional needs, taking into consideration any dietary restrictions or preferences such as low-carb, gluten-free, or plant-based diets. This foundational understanding will guide your choices and empower you to create meals that are both satisfying and conducive to your health goals.

When designing your weekly meal plan, focus on incorporating a variety of foods from different food groups. A Mediterranean diet, for example, emphasizes whole grains, lean proteins, healthy fats, and plenty of fruits and vegetables, making it an excellent framework for diabetic meal planning. Aim to include at least five servings of vegetables and three servings of fruits throughout the week. This not only provides essential vitamins and minerals but also adds fiber, which is beneficial for blood sugar control.

Another key aspect of meal planning is portion control. Using measuring cups or a food scale can help you understand serving sizes, ensuring you consume appropriate portions of carbohydrates, proteins, and fats. Consider creating balanced meals that consist of a source of protein, healthy fats, and complex carbohydrates. For instance, pairing grilled chicken with quinoa and a side of roasted vegetables provides a nutrient-dense meal that supports stable blood sugar levels while offering variety and flavor.

In addition to main meals, don't overlook the importance of snacks. Diabetic-friendly snack options can be both delicious and nutritious. Incorporate items such as hummus with vegetable sticks, Greek yogurt with berries, or a handful of nuts. These snacks can help bridge the gap between meals, maintain energy levels, and prevent drastic fluctuations in blood sugar. Planning these snacks in advance ensures that you have convenient and healthy options readily available.

Finally, consider meal prepping as part of your weekly planning. Preparing meals in advance not only saves time during busy weekdays but also helps you resist the temptation of unhealthy choices. Dedicate a few hours each week to batch-cook meals, portion them into containers, and store them in the refrigerator or freezer. This strategy can be particularly effective for managing portion sizes and ensuring that your meals align with your dietary goals. By investing time in planning and prepping, you lay the groundwork for a successful week of healthy eating.

Storage and Reheating Tips

When managing diabetes, proper storage and reheating of meals can significantly impact both the nutritional integrity and safety of the food.

To ensure that meals retain their quality, it is important to follow specific guidelines for storage. First, always allow cooked food to cool at room temperature for no more than two hours before refrigerating or freezing.

This practice prevents the growth of harmful bacteria. Utilize airtight containers to store meals, as they help maintain freshness while minimizing exposure to air, which can lead to spoilage. Label each container with the date it was prepared to keep track of freshness and ensure that you consume meals within their safe time frames.

When considering reheating, it is vital to do so in a way that preserves the nutritional value of the food. For best results, use a microwave or an oven rather than a stovetop, as these methods allow for more even heating. If using a microwave, cover the food with a microwave-safe lid or wrap to retain moisture, which can help maintain texture and flavor. Stirring the food halfway through reheating can also promote even heating. For those following a plant-based or Mediterranean diet, reheating meals can enhance flavors as ingredients meld together over time, making it an enjoyable experience.

Maintaining the integrity of specific components in diabetic-friendly meals, such as low-carb ingredients and gluten-free options, requires attention to detail when reheating. For example, whole grains or legumes can dry out during reheating, so adding a splash of water or broth can help restore moisture. Similarly, diabetic-friendly snacks, particularly those that are high in fiber, can benefit from a brief reheat to improve texture. Additionally, be cautious with reheating certain foods multiple times, as this can lead to nutrient loss, especially in vegetables that are rich in vitamins.

In terms of meal prep strategies, batch cooking can be an effective approach to managing a diabetic diet. Prepare larger quantities of meals and appropriately portion them into individual servings for quick access throughout the week. This practice not only saves time but also helps maintain a variety of options in your diet. When it comes to snacks, preparing healthy, diabetic-friendly options in advance can curb the temptation to reach for less nutritious choices. Store these snacks in easily accessible locations, ensuring they remain a convenient choice for in-between meals.

Lastly, for those incorporating intermittent fasting into their diabetes management plan, proper storage and reheating are crucial for adhering to eating windows. Meals should be prepared in advance to ensure they are ready to eat during designated eating times. Consider using a meal planner that allows for easy tracking of what has been prepared and when it should be consumed. By following these storage and reheating tips, individuals can optimize their meal preparation efforts, ensuring that their diabetic diet remains both enjoyable and beneficial to their overall health.

Chapter 13: Diabetes-Friendly Desserts

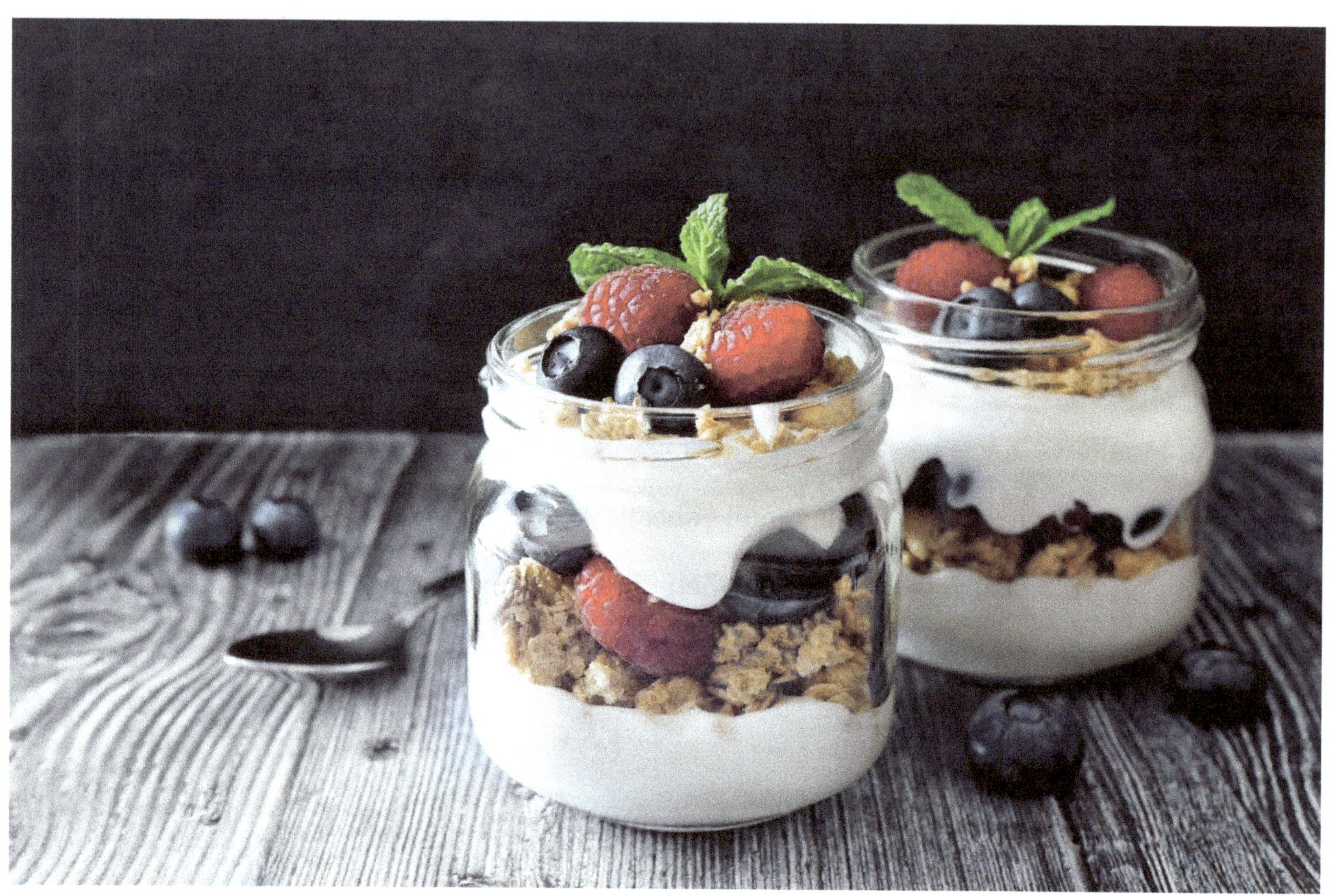

Indulgence Without Guilt

Indulgence without guilt is a concept that resonates deeply with those managing diabetes, as the journey often involves navigating cravings while adhering to dietary restrictions. The good news is that enjoying delicious meals and snacks does not have to come at the expense of health. By embracing flavors and ingredients that align with a diabetic-friendly lifestyle, individuals can craft a diet that is not only satisfying but also nourishing. This balance is essential in fostering a positive relationship with food while managing blood sugar levels effectively.

Incorporating low-carb options into your diet can pave the way for indulgence without compromising health. By focusing on whole, unprocessed foods, you can create meals that are rich in flavor yet low in carbohydrates. For example, zucchini noodles or cauliflower rice can serve as excellent substitutes for traditional pasta and rice. These alternatives not only provide a satisfying texture but also allow for a variety of sauces and toppings that can elevate your meals. By experimenting with herbs and spices, you can enhance the taste of these dishes, making them feel indulgent while keeping your carbohydrate intake in check.

Plant-based diets offer another avenue for enjoying food without guilt. Incorporating more vegetables, legumes, nuts, and seeds into your meals can provide essential nutrients while allowing for creative culinary exploration. Dishes like lentil curry or roasted vegetable salads can be both filling and flavorful. Additionally, plant-based recipes often align with the principles of the Mediterranean diet, which emphasizes healthy fats, whole grains, and a variety of colorful produce. This not only supports blood sugar management but also contributes to overall well-being.

For those with a sweet tooth, diabetic-friendly desserts can satisfy cravings without the worry of spikes in blood sugar. Utilizing natural sweeteners like stevia or monk fruit, along with ingredients such as almond flour or coconut flour, allows for the creation of treats that are both delicious and compatible with a diabetic diet.

Recipes for chia seed puddings, fruit-based sorbets, or dark chocolate treats can provide the indulgence one desires while still adhering to dietary guidelines. These options demonstrate that desserts need not be a guilty pleasure but rather a delightful component of a balanced diet.

Finally, the concept of indulgence extends to snacks, which often serve as a bridge between meals. Choosing snacks that are high in protein and fiber, such as Greek yogurt with berries or hummus with vegetables, can help maintain steady blood sugar levels while still providing satisfaction. Planning and preparing diabetic-friendly snacks in advance can make it easier to indulge mindfully without reaching for processed options that may not align with your dietary goals. By embracing these strategies, individuals can enjoy a variety of foods while maintaining control over their health, proving that indulgence and a healthy lifestyle can coexist harmoniously.

Healthy Dessert Recipes

Healthy desserts can be a delightful addition to any diabetic diet, proving that indulgence doesn't have to come at the cost of health. With the right ingredients and a focus on lower-carb options, it is possible to create satisfying treats that align with diabetic nutritional guidelines. The key lies in using natural sweeteners, whole ingredients, and incorporating fiber-rich components that help stabilize blood sugar levels. This approach allows individuals to enjoy desserts without compromising their health goals.

One popular option is to use almond flour or coconut flour as a base for baked goods. These flours are low in carbohydrates and high in fiber, making them excellent substitutes for traditional wheat flour. Recipes for almond flour cookies or coconut flour brownies can satisfy sweet cravings while providing the necessary nutrients without spiking blood sugar levels. Additionally, incorporating ingredients like unsweetened cocoa powder can enhance flavor while also delivering antioxidants.

Fruits can also serve as a natural sweetener in desserts. Berries, such as strawberries, blueberries, and raspberries, are not only low in sugar but also rich in vitamins and minerals. A simple berry parfait made with Greek yogurt can be an excellent choice for a diabetic-friendly dessert. By layering fresh berries with a dollop of yogurt and a sprinkle of nuts, one can create a visually appealing and nutritious dessert that is both satisfying and healthy.

Another approach to healthy desserts is to explore the use of plant-based ingredients. Desserts made from ingredients like avocados, bananas, or sweet potatoes can provide creamy textures and natural sweetness. For example, a chocolate avocado mousse harnesses the healthy fats from avocados while delivering a rich chocolate flavor. This dessert not only satisfies chocolate cravings but also provides essential nutrients that support overall health and wellness.

Finally, incorporating spices such as cinnamon or vanilla can enhance the flavor of desserts without adding extra sugar. These spices can elevate the taste of baked goods, smoothies, or even chia seed puddings. By focusing on whole food ingredients and mindful cooking methods, individuals can enjoy a variety of healthy dessert recipes that support their dietary needs while still allowing for moments of sweetness and indulgence.

Substitutions for Traditional Sweets

In the quest for maintaining a balanced diabetic diet, the craving for traditional sweets can pose a challenge. However, there are numerous substitutions that can satisfy those sweet cravings without compromising health. Understanding the role of ingredients and their impact on blood sugar levels is essential for anyone managing diabetes. By making informed choices, individuals can enjoy delicious alternatives that not only taste good but also align with dietary needs.

One popular substitution for traditional sweets is the use of natural sweeteners like stevia, monk fruit, and erythritol. These sugar alternatives provide sweetness without causing significant spikes in blood glucose levels. Stevia, derived from the leaves of the Stevia plant, is a zero-calorie sweetener that can be used in baking, beverages, and sauces. Monk fruit extract, another natural option, offers a sweet flavor profile without the calories or carbohydrates found in conventional sugar. Erythritol, a sugar alcohol, contains minimal calories and is well-tolerated, making it an excellent choice for sweetening desserts and snacks.

Incorporating fruits into desserts can also serve as a healthful substitution. Fresh berries, for instance, are low in carbohydrates and high in fiber, making them an ideal choice for a diabetic-friendly sweet treat. Blending fruits like bananas or avocados into smoothies can create a creamy, sweet base without the need for added sugars. Additionally, using pureed fruits in place of sugar in baking can enhance flavor while reducing calorie content. The natural sweetness from fruits, combined with their nutritional benefits, makes them a valuable component of a diabetic diet.

Another effective strategy is to explore recipes that utilize whole grains and nuts in place of refined flours and sugars. Almond flour, coconut flour, and oat flour can be used to create low-carb baked goods that are both satisfying and nutritious. These alternatives provide essential nutrients and healthy fats, contributing to satiety and stable blood sugar levels. Incorporating ingredients such as unsweetened cocoa powder or dark chocolate can also enhance the flavor profile of desserts while minimizing sugar content. These swaps allow for the creation of indulgent treats without the adverse effects on health.

Lastly, the Mediterranean diet offers a wealth of options for those seeking diabetic-friendly sweets. Traditional Mediterranean desserts often emphasize nuts, seeds, and fruits, which provide healthy fats and fiber. Items like baklava can be adapted using nut-based crusts and natural sweeteners, creating a guilt-free version of this classic treat. Yogurt parfaits layered with fresh fruits and nuts can serve as a delightful dessert while promoting gut health. By embracing the principles of the Mediterranean diet, individuals can discover a variety of culturally specific sweets that align with their dietary requirements.

In conclusion, with thoughtful substitutions and ingredient choices, it is entirely possible to enjoy satisfying sweets while managing diabetes. By utilizing natural sweeteners, incorporating fruits, opting for whole grains, and exploring Mediterranean-inspired recipes, individuals can indulge their sweet tooth without compromising their health. These strategies not only enhance the enjoyment of food but also support a balanced and nutritious approach to diabetes management.

Chapter 14:
Culturally Specific Diabetic Diets

Exploring Global Diets

Exploring global diets reveals a wealth of culinary traditions that can cater to the needs of individuals managing diabetes. Different cultures have developed unique dietary practices that not only reflect their history and environment but also provide valuable insights into maintaining balanced nutrition. These diets often emphasize whole foods, seasonal ingredients, and portion control, making them suitable for those seeking to manage their blood sugar levels effectively. By examining various global diets, individuals can discover new ways to diversify their meal plans while adhering to diabetic-friendly guidelines.

The Mediterranean diet stands out as a prime example of a nutritious approach to eating that is beneficial for diabetics. Rich in vegetables, fruits, whole grains, legumes, nuts, and healthy fats, this diet focuses on the consumption of unprocessed foods, which can help stabilize blood sugar levels. Olive oil serves as the primary fat source, providing monounsaturated fats that are heart-healthy and anti-inflammatory. Additionally, the inclusion of fish and lean meats in moderation supports a balanced intake of protein while minimizing saturated fats. Adopting principles from the Mediterranean diet can lead to improved overall health and better diabetes management.

Plant-based diets also offer a compelling option for those managing diabetes. By centering meals around whole plant foods such as vegetables, fruits, legumes, grains, nuts, and seeds, individuals can enhance their fiber intake, which is beneficial for blood sugar control.

The high fiber content in these foods helps slow digestion and promotes satiety, reducing the likelihood of blood sugar spikes. Furthermore, plant-based diets are often low in saturated fats and cholesterol, making them heart-healthy choices for diabetics. Exploring plant-based recipes can inspire creativity in the kitchen while adhering to dietary restrictions.

Culturally specific diets provide another avenue for exploring diabetes-friendly eating patterns. Many traditional diets around the world have natural components that align with diabetic needs. For instance, Asian diets often emphasize rice, vegetables, and fish, while Latin American diets include a variety of beans, corn, and fresh produce. Understanding these cultural nuances allows individuals to adapt traditional recipes to fit their dietary requirements, fostering a sense of connection to their heritage while prioritizing health. By incorporating elements from various global cuisines, individuals can enjoy diverse flavors and textures in their meals.

In addition to meal composition, successful diabetes management also involves strategic planning and preparation. Intermittent fasting has gained popularity as a method to help regulate blood sugar levels and promote weight management. By structuring eating windows, individuals can better control their caloric intake and potentially enhance insulin sensitivity. Meal prep strategies tailored for diabetics can simplify the process of adhering to dietary guidelines, ensuring that healthy, balanced meals and snacks are readily available. By integrating the principles of global diets with practical meal prep techniques, individuals can cultivate a sustainable and enjoyable approach to managing their diabetes.

Adapting Traditional Recipes

Adapting traditional recipes is an essential skill for anyone managing diabetes, as it allows individuals to enjoy beloved dishes while adhering to dietary restrictions. Many traditional recipes are rich in carbohydrates and sugars, which can pose challenges for blood sugar management. However, with a creative approach, these recipes can be modified to fit a diabetic-friendly lifestyle without sacrificing flavor or cultural significance. By focusing on ingredient substitutions and cooking techniques, individuals can reclaim their favorite meals.

One effective strategy for adapting traditional recipes is to replace high-carb ingredients with lower-carb alternatives. For example, in pasta dishes, consider using spiralized vegetables such as zucchini or spaghetti squash instead of traditional pasta. Cauliflower rice can serve as a great substitute for regular rice in dishes like stir-fries or risottos. These swaps not only reduce the carbohydrate content but also add nutritional benefits, such as increased fiber and vitamins, which are essential for overall health.

In addition to ingredient substitutions, altering cooking methods can significantly impact the nutritional profile of traditional recipes. Techniques such as grilling, steaming, or baking can replace frying, resulting in dishes that are lower in unhealthy fats. For instance, instead of deep-frying traditional favorites like eggplant or chicken, try baking them with a light coating of olive oil and herbs for a healthier twist. This not only preserves the flavor but also aligns with the principles of the Mediterranean diet, which emphasizes healthy fats and whole foods.

Culturally specific diets can also provide a foundation for creating diabetic-friendly adaptations. By focusing on the core elements of these cuisines, one can maintain authenticity while ensuring that the dishes meet dietary needs. For instance, in Mexican cuisine, traditional rice and beans can be modified by using black beans in moderation and pairing them with a larger portion of non-starchy vegetables. This approach keeps the meal satisfying while balancing blood sugar levels effectively.

Finally, the incorporation of diabetic-friendly snacks and desserts is crucial in adapting traditional recipes. Many traditional sweets can be modified using natural sweeteners like stevia or erythritol, which have minimal impact on blood sugar levels. Furthermore, adding ingredients such as nuts, seeds, and yogurt can enrich snacks while providing essential nutrients.

By embracing these adaptations, individuals can enjoy a diverse array of flavors and textures that support their health goals, making the journey of managing diabetes both enjoyable and sustainable.

Cultural Considerations in Meal Planning

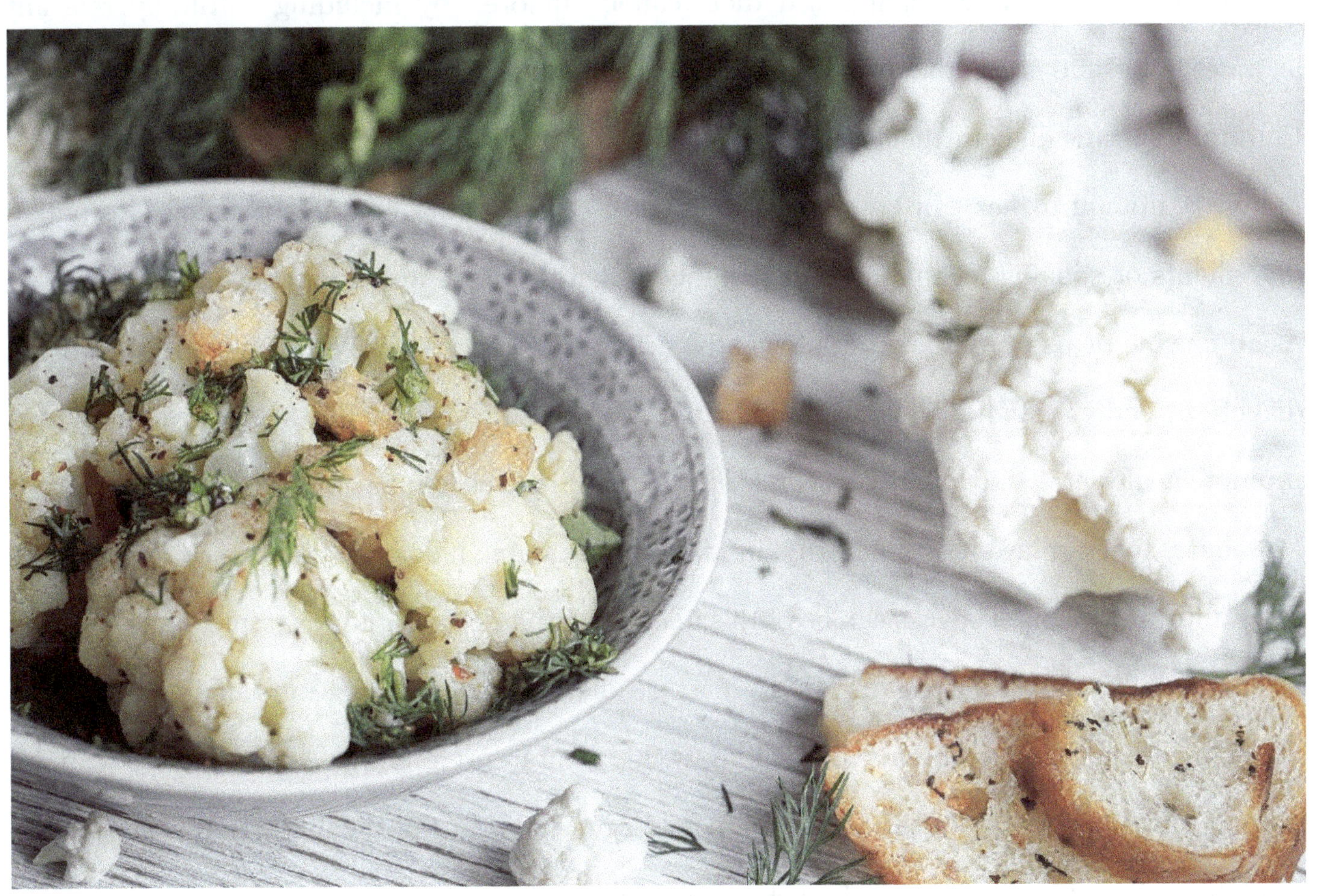

Cultural considerations play a pivotal role in meal planning, particularly for individuals managing diabetes. Understanding the cultural significance of various foods helps in creating meal plans that are not only nutritious but also respectful of traditional eating habits. Each culture has its unique culinary practices, flavors, and ingredients that can be adapted to fit a diabetic-friendly framework. By recognizing these cultural nuances, meal planning can be more inclusive and appealing, which is essential for long-term adherence to dietary changes.

Incorporating traditional foods into diabetic meal plans can enhance the enjoyment of eating while still adhering to nutritional guidelines. For example, Mediterranean diets, which emphasize whole grains, vegetables, lean proteins, and healthy fats, can be modified to accommodate low-carb preferences without sacrificing flavor. Utilizing herbs and spices common in Mediterranean cuisine can elevate dishes without the need for added sugars or unhealthy fats. Similarly, plant-based diets can be tailored by including culturally relevant legumes, nuts, and grains that provide necessary nutrients while aiding in blood sugar control.

Culturally specific diabetic diets also require attention to portion sizes and preparation methods. Many traditional dishes can be adapted to reduce carbohydrate content by using alternative ingredients or cooking techniques. For instance, substituting white rice with cauliflower rice in Asian cuisine or using whole grain alternatives in Latin American recipes can create healthier, diabetic-friendly options. These modifications not only respect cultural heritage but also promote healthier eating habits that can lead to better diabetes management.

Moreover, snacks play an essential role in maintaining stable blood sugar levels throughout the day. Culturally inspired snacks can be both satisfying and nutritious. For example, incorporating hummus with vegetable sticks in Middle Eastern diets or using spiced nuts in Indian cuisine offers diabetes-friendly options that align with cultural preferences. These snacks can be prepared in advance as part of a meal prep strategy, ensuring that healthy choices are always available, which can prevent impulsive eating of high-carb or sugary foods.

Lastly, it's essential to consider nutritional supplements within the context of cultural diets. Some cultures may rely on specific foods that are rich in particular vitamins or minerals, which can complement a diabetic diet effectively. Understanding the role of these foods allows for the incorporation of supplements where necessary, ensuring that nutritional needs are met without compromising cultural identity. By blending cultural considerations with diabetes management strategies, individuals can enjoy a diverse and fulfilling diet that supports their health goals.

Chapter 15: Nutritional Supplements for Diabetics

Overview of Common Supplements

In the realm of diabetes management, nutritional supplements play a pivotal role in supporting overall health and addressing specific dietary needs. Individuals managing diabetes often seek ways to enhance their nutritional intake while adhering to dietary restrictions. Common supplements such as vitamins, minerals, and herbal extracts can provide additional benefits that complement a balanced diet, particularly for those following specific meal plans like low-carb, Mediterranean, or plant-based diets. Understanding these supplements and their potential contributions can empower individuals to make informed choices that align with their health goals.

One of the most frequently utilized supplements for diabetics is chromium, a mineral that may aid in improving insulin sensitivity. Research suggests that chromium can help regulate blood sugar levels, making it a valuable addition for those striving to maintain glycemic control. Additionally, magnesium plays a crucial role in carbohydrate metabolism and has been linked to better blood sugar regulation. Many diabetic meal plans may lack sufficient magnesium due to dietary restrictions, highlighting the importance of considering this supplement for individuals aiming to enhance their nutritional status.

Omega-3 fatty acids are another supplement worth considering, particularly for those interested in heart health alongside diabetes management. Found in fish oil and certain plant-based sources like flaxseed, omega-3s have demonstrated anti-inflammatory properties and potential cardiovascular benefits.

For individuals following a Mediterranean or plant-based diet, incorporating omega-3 supplements can help achieve the recommended intake, particularly in the absence of fatty fish. This can be especially beneficial for men and women who prioritize heart health in their diabetes management strategies.

Vitamin D and B-complex vitamins also deserve attention in the context of diabetic nutrition. Vitamin D deficiency is common among individuals with diabetes, and supplementation may improve insulin sensitivity and overall metabolic health. Similarly, B vitamins, particularly B12 and folate, are essential for energy metabolism and neurological function. For those on gluten-free diets or specific meal plans that may inadvertently reduce B vitamin intake, supplementation can help bridge potential gaps in nutrition, ensuring that individuals meet their dietary needs.

Finally, herbal supplements such as berberine and cinnamon have gained popularity for their potential blood sugar-lowering effects. Both have shown promise in studies for improving insulin sensitivity and aiding in glycemic control. Incorporating these supplements into a diabetic-friendly diet can provide an additional layer of support, particularly for individuals exploring low-carb or culturally specific dietary approaches.

However, it is essential to consult healthcare professionals before starting any new supplement regimen to ensure safety and compatibility with existing health conditions and medications.

Benefits and Risks

The management of diabetes through dietary choices presents both notable benefits and inherent risks that must be carefully navigated. A well-structured diabetic diet can lead to improved blood sugar control, weight management, and overall health. For individuals adhering to low-carb meal plans, the restricted intake of carbohydrates helps to stabilize glucose levels, reducing the risk of spikes and crashes. Additionally, plant-based diets can enhance fiber intake, which is crucial for digestive health and can aid in regulating blood sugar levels. Adopting the Mediterranean diet, rich in healthy fats and antioxidants, may also offer protective benefits against cardiovascular complications often associated with diabetes.

However, the benefits of these diets must be weighed against potential risks. For example, individuals who significantly reduce their carbohydrate intake may experience nutrient deficiencies if they do not carefully plan their meals. It's essential for those following a low-carb or gluten-free diet to ensure they are still receiving adequate vitamins and minerals from alternative sources. Moreover, while the Mediterranean diet can be highly beneficial, overconsumption of high-calorie foods, even if they are healthy fats, can lead to weight gain. As with any dietary approach, moderation and balance are key to avoiding adverse effects.

Incorporating diabetic-friendly snacks into one's diet can provide a convenient way to maintain energy levels and prevent hunger pangs, yet the selection of these snacks warrants scrutiny. Many commercially available options may contain hidden sugars or unhealthy fats that could undermine blood sugar control. Homemade snacks, on the other hand, allow for greater control over ingredients and portion sizes. This proactive approach can enhance the effectiveness of a diabetic diet but requires planning and preparation, which can be an added challenge for some individuals.

Intermittent fasting has emerged as a popular strategy for diabetes management, with research suggesting it may improve insulin sensitivity and promote weight loss. However, this approach is not suitable for everyone and can pose risks for individuals who may experience hypoglycemia or other complications. It is crucial for those considering intermittent fasting to consult healthcare professionals to tailor the plan to their specific needs and health status. Understanding one's body and its reactions to various eating patterns is essential to harnessing the benefits while minimizing risks.

Finally, nutritional supplements may offer additional support for those managing diabetes, yet they should complement, not replace, a healthy diet. The unregulated nature of many supplements raises concerns about their efficacy and safety. It is advisable for individuals to seek guidance from healthcare providers before incorporating supplements into their routine, ensuring they align with their dietary goals and medical needs. By being informed and cautious, individuals can enjoy the benefits of a diabetic diet while mitigating risks, leading to a healthier, more balanced lifestyle.

Consulting with Healthcare Providers

Consulting with healthcare providers is a critical step in managing diabetes effectively. When embarking on a diabetic diet, it is essential for individuals to work closely with a variety of healthcare professionals, including doctors, registered dietitians, and diabetes educators. Each of these experts plays a vital role in tailoring dietary recommendations to meet individual health needs while ensuring that nutritional choices align with medical guidelines. Open communication with healthcare providers can help in developing a comprehensive meal plan that considers personal preferences and lifestyle.

One of the first steps in this consultation is to assess individual health conditions, including comorbidities that may influence dietary choices. For example, individuals with diabetes may also have hypertension or high cholesterol, necessitating a multifaceted approach to food selection. Healthcare providers can help identify specific dietary patterns such as low-carb, plant-based, or Mediterranean diets, which have been shown to support better blood sugar control. They can also provide guidance on gluten-free options for those with celiac disease or gluten sensitivity, ensuring that all meals are both safe and beneficial.

A significant aspect of consulting with healthcare providers is the ongoing education about diabetes management. This includes understanding the impact of various foods on glucose levels and learning to read nutrition labels effectively. Dietitians can offer insights into portion control and meal timing, which are crucial for those interested in intermittent fasting as a strategy for blood sugar regulation. By engaging in discussions about food choices and their implications, individuals can develop a deeper understanding of how their diet affects their overall health.

Healthcare providers can also assist in identifying suitable diabetic-friendly snack options and desserts that align with dietary restrictions. They can recommend recipes and meal prep strategies that simplify the cooking process while ensuring meals are nutritious and enjoyable. Culturally specific diets may also be explored, allowing individuals to maintain their culinary traditions while adhering to diabetic guidelines. This personalized approach not only promotes better adherence to dietary recommendations but also enhances the overall quality of life.

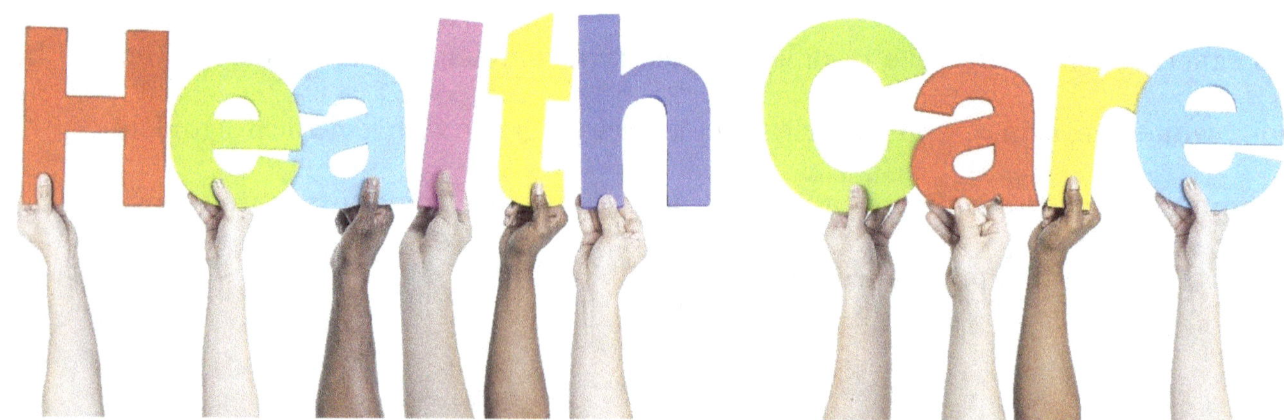

Lastly, consulting with healthcare providers should include discussions about the use of nutritional supplements. While a well-balanced diet is the cornerstone of diabetes management, certain individuals may benefit from supplements to address specific deficiencies or enhance overall well-being. Providers can help determine the appropriateness of supplements based on individual health assessments and dietary intake. This collaborative effort fosters a holistic approach to diabetes care, empowering individuals to take charge of their health through informed dietary choices.

Chapter 16:
Creating a Sustainable Lifestyle

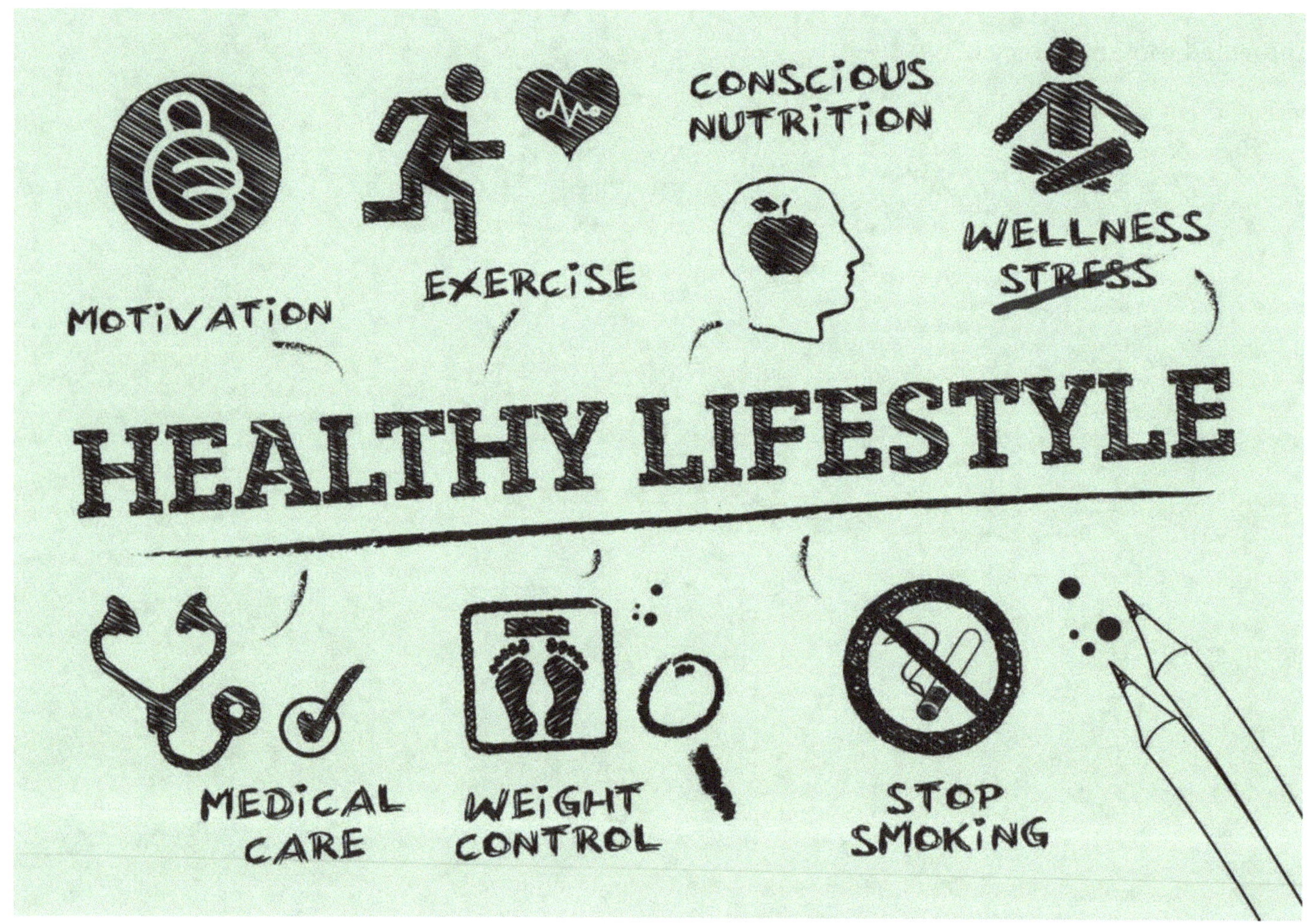

Building Healthy Habits

Building healthy habits is essential for managing diabetes effectively and maintaining overall well-being. For both men and women navigating the complexities of a diabetic diet, establishing consistent routines can significantly impact blood sugar levels and health outcomes.

The foundation of these habits begins with understanding the principles of a balanced diet tailored to individual needs, such as low-carb meal plans and plant-based options. By integrating these dietary elements into daily life, individuals can feel empowered to make healthier choices that align with their diabetes management goals.

A fundamental aspect of building healthy habits is meal planning. Creating structured meal plans that include diabetic-friendly recipes can simplify grocery shopping and cooking while ensuring that nutritional needs are met. This approach allows for the inclusion of Mediterranean diet principles, which emphasize whole foods, healthy fats, and lean proteins. By planning meals ahead of time, individuals can avoid impulsive food choices that may not support their health objectives. Additionally, incorporating gluten-free recipes ensures that those with sensitivities can still enjoy a diverse and satisfying diet.

Incorporating healthy snacks into daily routines is another vital strategy. Diabetic-friendly snacks can help manage hunger between meals while stabilizing blood sugar levels. Options such as nuts, seeds, and fresh fruits are not only nutritious but also easily portable, making them ideal for busy lifestyles. By keeping these snacks readily available, individuals can resist the temptation of less healthy alternatives when cravings arise. Developing a repertoire of go-to snacks will bolster the habit of mindful eating and support better blood sugar management.

Intermittent fasting is another practice that has gained popularity for diabetes control. This approach allows individuals to structure their eating patterns in a way that supports metabolic health. By creating designated windows for eating, individuals can improve insulin sensitivity and reduce the overall caloric intake without feeling deprived.

It is essential, however, to ensure that meals consumed during eating windows are balanced and provide the necessary nutrients for maintaining energy levels. As with any dietary strategy, it is crucial to consult healthcare professionals before making significant changes.

Finally, cultural considerations play an important role in building healthy habits. Culturally specific diabetic diets can provide familiar and satisfying meal options while adhering to health guidelines. Engaging with traditional foods and recipes can enhance the sustainability of dietary changes, making healthy eating feel less like a restriction and more like an enjoyable lifestyle. Additionally, exploring nutritional supplements may enhance the overall dietary plan, providing essential nutrients that support diabetes management. By focusing on these diverse aspects of diet and lifestyle, individuals can cultivate healthy habits that promote long-term health and well-being.

Staying Motivated

Staying motivated while managing a diabetic diet can be a challenging endeavor, particularly given the numerous dietary restrictions and lifestyle changes involved. It is essential to recognize that motivation is not a constant state; it fluctuates and evolves. To stay on track, begin by setting realistic and achievable goals. Instead of aiming for drastic changes overnight, focus on small, incremental adjustments that can lead to sustainable habits. Celebrate each achievement, whether
it's successfully preparing a diabetic-friendly meal or resisting the temptation of unhealthy snacks. This positive reinforcement can significantly enhance your motivation.

Another crucial aspect of maintaining motivation is education. Understanding the impact of different foods on blood sugar levels allows individuals to make informed choices. Familiarize yourself with the principles of a low-carb meal plan or the benefits of a Mediterranean diet tailored for diabetes management. Knowledge of how specific ingredients can optimize health will empower you to create meals that are not only compliant with dietary needs but also enjoyable. This understanding can transform the experience of meal preparation from a chore into a creative and fulfilling process.

Incorporating variety into your diet is another effective way to stay motivated. A diverse menu can prevent the monotony that often leads to boredom and, ultimately, abandonment of dietary goals. Explore the world of plant-based recipes, gluten-free options, and culturally specific dishes that align with diabetic dietary needs. Experimenting with new flavors and textures can reignite your enthusiasm for cooking and eating, making each meal something to look forward to. Furthermore, engaging in meal prep strategies can simplify the process, ensuring that you always have healthy options readily available.

Community support plays a vital role in sustaining motivation in any lifestyle change, including dietary management for diabetes. Surrounding yourself with individuals who understand your journey can provide encouragement and accountability. Whether through online forums, local support groups, or social media, sharing experiences, recipes, and challenges with others can foster a sense of belonging. Additionally, consider involving friends and family in your meal preparation and dining experiences, making it a collective endeavor that enhances your motivation and reinforces healthy habits.

Lastly, remember to be kind to yourself throughout this process. Managing diabetes is a lifelong commitment that comes with its ups and downs. It is normal to encounter setbacks, whether it is indulging in a dessert or veering off your meal plan. Rather than allowing guilt to diminish your motivation, view these moments as learning opportunities. Reflect on what led to the choice and how you can adjust your approach moving forward. Embracing a flexible mindset will help you stay committed to your goals while enjoying the journey of discovering a healthier, diabetic-friendly lifestyle.

Long-Term Strategies for Success

Long-term success in managing diabetes through diet requires a multifaceted approach that goes beyond temporary changes. Adopting a sustainable diabetic meal plan is crucial for maintaining stable blood sugar levels and overall health. This involves selecting appropriate food groups, understanding portion control, and incorporating a variety of nutrients into daily meals. A well-rounded diet that includes low-carb options, plant-based foods, and Mediterranean influences can significantly improve glycemic control. It is essential to make informed choices that align with personal preferences and cultural practices, ensuring that the diet remains enjoyable and fulfilling.

Incorporating meal prep strategies can be a game changer for individuals managing diabetes. Preparing meals in advance not only saves time during busy weekdays but also helps in making healthier choices. Planning weekly menus with diabetic-friendly recipes allows for better control over ingredients and portion sizes. Consideration of gluten-free options can also be beneficial for those with sensitivities, ensuring that meals are both safe and nutritious. By organizing meals ahead of time, individuals can avoid impulsive decisions that may lead to unhealthy eating patterns.

Intermittent fasting emerges as another effective strategy for long-term success in diabetes management. This approach can help regulate insulin sensitivity and improve metabolic health. Research suggests that intermittent fasting may aid in weight management, a critical component for many individuals managing diabetes. However, it is important to approach this eating pattern cautiously, ensuring that meals consumed during non-fasting periods are balanced and nutritious. Consulting with a healthcare provider can help tailor this strategy to fit individual health needs and lifestyle preferences.

Finding satisfying and diabetes-friendly snack options is essential for maintaining energy levels and preventing blood sugar spikes. Snacking can be a vital part of the daily routine, and choosing snacks that are low in carbohydrates and high in fiber can help keep blood sugar levels stable. Options such as raw vegetables with hummus, nuts, or Greek yogurt can be both delicious and beneficial. Exploring culturally specific snacks that align with diabetic guidelines can also enhance dietary adherence and enjoyment, making it easier to maintain a healthy lifestyle.

Finally, incorporating nutritional supplements can play a supportive role in a diabetic diet. Supplements such as omega-3 fatty acids, magnesium, and vitamin D may offer additional health benefits, improving overall well-being and aiding in diabetes management. However, it is crucial to consult healthcare professionals before adding any supplements to ensure they complement dietary choices and do not interfere with medications. By integrating these long-term strategies into daily life, individuals can create a sustainable, enjoyable, and effective approach to managing diabetes through diet.

Chapter 17:
Meal Prep for Special Occasions

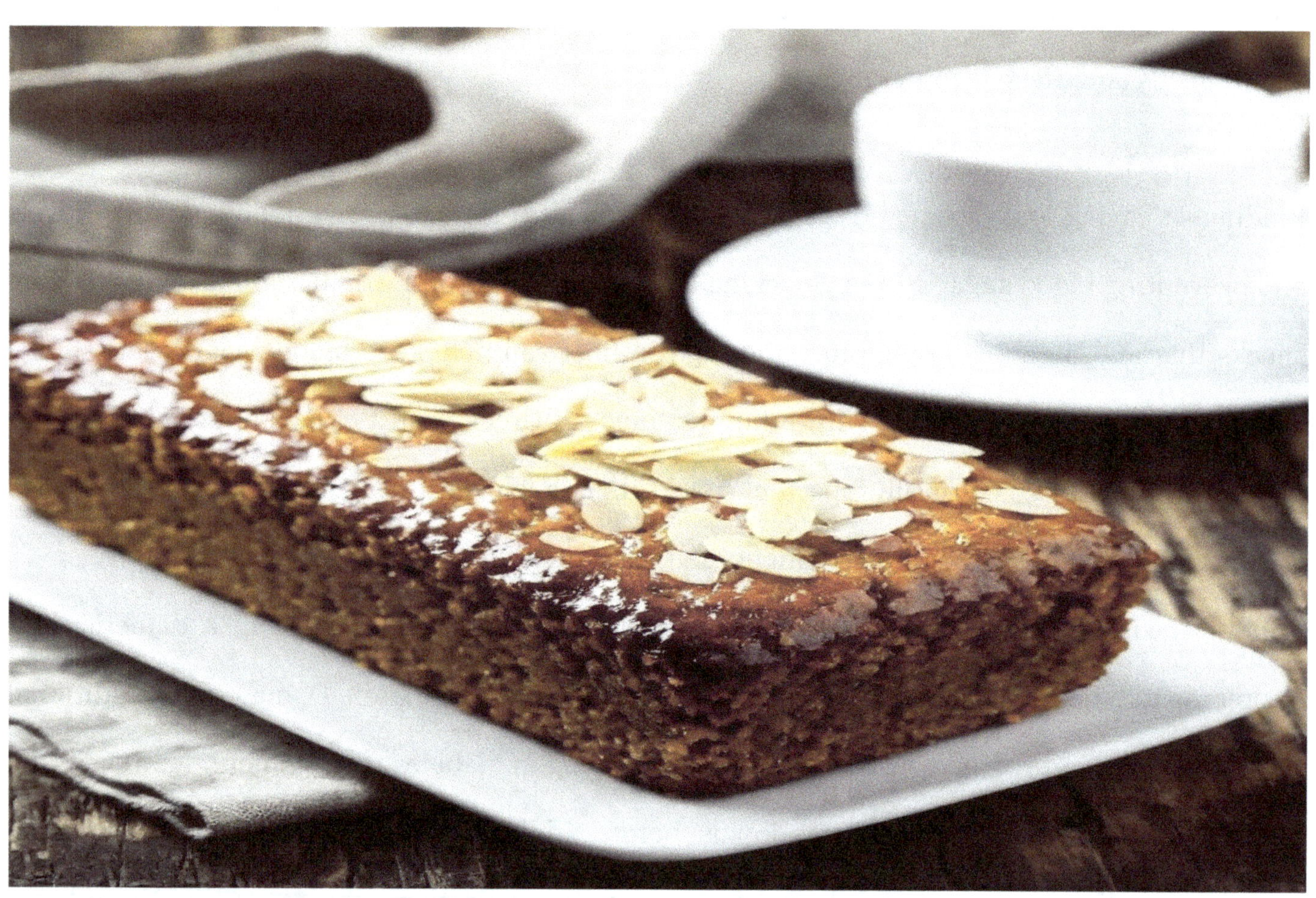

Healthy Holiday Recipes

Healthy holiday recipes can be a delightful way to celebrate seasonal festivities while adhering to dietary restrictions associated with diabetes. This subchapter presents a selection of nutritious, low-carb, and diabetic-friendly recipes that cater to various palates and cultural preferences.

By incorporating whole foods, fresh vegetables, and lean proteins, these recipes are designed to promote health and well-being during the holiday season.

For starters, consider a Mediterranean-inspired roasted vegetable platter. Utilizing seasonal vegetables like zucchini, bell peppers, and eggplant, this dish is not only visually appealing but also rich in fiber and low in carbohydrates. Drizzle the vegetables with olive oil, sprinkle with fresh herbs such as oregano and thyme, and roast them until tender. This colorful appetizer is perfect for sharing and offers a satisfying option that aligns with diabetic dietary guidelines.

Another excellent addition to your holiday table could be a plant-based lentil salad. Lentils are an excellent source of protein and fiber, helping to stabilize blood sugar levels. Combine cooked lentils with diced cucumbers, cherry tomatoes, red onion, and parsley, then dress with a lemon vinaigrette. This refreshing salad can serve as a main dish or a side, making it versatile enough for any holiday gathering. Its vibrant flavors and textures will impress guests while keeping their health in mind.

For those looking for diabetic-friendly snacks, consider creating a cheese and nut platter. Select a variety of low-fat cheeses and pair them with unsalted nuts like almonds and walnuts. Add some fresh fruit, such as sliced apples or berries, to balance the flavors without overwhelming blood sugar levels. This combination not only provides healthy fats and protein but also offers a satisfying crunch and sweetness that can curb holiday cravings.

Lastly, desserts can also be made diabetic-friendly without sacrificing taste. A sugar-free pumpkin pie made with almond flour crust and sweetened with a sugar substitute is a perfect example. This recipe allows you to enjoy the traditional flavors of the season while controlling carbohydrate intake. Serve it with a dollop of whipped coconut cream for an indulgent yet health-conscious treat that everyone can enjoy, making the holidays enjoyable for those managing diabetes.

Family Gatherings and Potlucks

Family gatherings and potlucks are cherished occasions that provide an opportunity to connect with loved ones while sharing delicious food. However, for those managing diabetes, these events can present challenges in maintaining dietary goals. It is essential to approach these gatherings with a strategy that allows participation without compromising health. Understanding how to navigate these social situations can help ensure that everyone enjoys the event while supporting their diabetes management.

When attending a potluck, consider bringing a diabetic-friendly dish that not only aligns with your dietary needs but also showcases the flavors and creativity of a nutritious meal. Options such as a Mediterranean quinoa salad, rich in plant-based ingredients, provide a vibrant, low-carb choice that is both filling and satisfying. This dish can easily accommodate various dietary preferences, making it a hit among family members. Including a variety of colorful vegetables and a light, homemade dressing can elevate the dish while keeping it diabetes-friendly.

Encouraging family members to contribute dishes that are considerate of diabetes can transform the gathering into a supportive environment. Sharing low-carb, gluten-free recipes not only fosters inclusivity but also educates others about the importance of healthy eating for diabetes management. When everyone participates in preparing meals that are both delicious and diabetic-friendly, it ensures that there are ample options available for those who need to be mindful of their carbohydrate intake.

In addition to main dishes, consider the importance of snacks at family gatherings. Diabetic-friendly snacks, such as vegetable trays with hummus or mixed nuts, can provide satisfying options that help to control blood sugar levels. These snacks not only cater to those managing diabetes but also appeal to a broader audience. Providing a selection of healthy choices encourages everyone to indulge without the guilt, creating a more enjoyable experience for all attendees.

Finally, desserts can still play a role in family gatherings without overwhelming your dietary restrictions. Explore diabetic-friendly dessert options that utilize natural sweeteners or are low in carbohydrates. Dishes like chia seed pudding or fruit salads made with a variety of berries can satisfy sweet cravings while being mindful of glucose levels. By incorporating these strategies into your family gatherings and potlucks, you can create an environment that celebrates health and togetherness while keeping diabetes management at the forefront.

Celebrating Birthdays and Anniversaries

Celebrating birthdays and anniversaries is a cherished tradition that brings people together, fostering joy and connection. However, for individuals managing diabetes, these celebrations can pose unique challenges, particularly when it comes to food choices. It is essential to approach these occasions with a mindset that prioritizes health while still allowing for indulgence.
By incorporating diabetic-friendly options, you can create memorable experiences that honor both the significance of the occasion and your dietary needs.

When planning a birthday or anniversary meal, consider the benefits of a low-carb diabetic meal plan. These plans not only help regulate blood sugar levels but also offer a variety of delicious options that can be enjoyed by all guests. Focus on incorporating lean proteins, healthy fats, and non-starchy vegetables into your main courses. For instance, grilled salmon paired with a vibrant Mediterranean salad can serve as a stunning centerpiece that is both satisfying and mindful of dietary restrictions.

Desserts often take center stage during celebrations, but they can be adapted to be diabetes-friendly without sacrificing flavor. Exploring plant-based and gluten-free recipes can lead to delightful alternatives that everyone can enjoy. Options such as chia seed pudding sweetened with natural sweeteners or almond flour cupcakes topped with a light cream cheese frosting or sugar-free almond and carrot cake provide a sweet touch that aligns with diabetic dietary guidelines. By emphasizing naturally sweet ingredients, these desserts can satisfy cravings while keeping blood sugar levels in check.

Snacking is another important aspect of celebrations, particularly during gatherings. Offering a selection of diabetic-friendly snacks can enhance the experience for all attendees. Consider serving a variety of colorful vegetable platters accompanied by hummus, or creating a cheese and nut board featuring heart-healthy options. These snacks not only cater to those managing diabetes but also promote a shared sense of health-conscious enjoyment that can resonate with everyone at the celebration.

Finally, incorporating intermittent fasting principles into your celebration can provide additional health benefits while still allowing for a festive atmosphere. By scheduling meal times thoughtfully and encouraging guests to partake in a balanced feast during designated eating windows, you can create an environment that supports diabetes management. Ultimately, celebrating birthdays and anniversaries does not have to be at odds with health; instead, it can be an opportunity to explore innovative, delicious, and nutritious options that bring people together in a meaningful way.

Chapter 18:
Staying Motivated on Your Meal Prep Journey

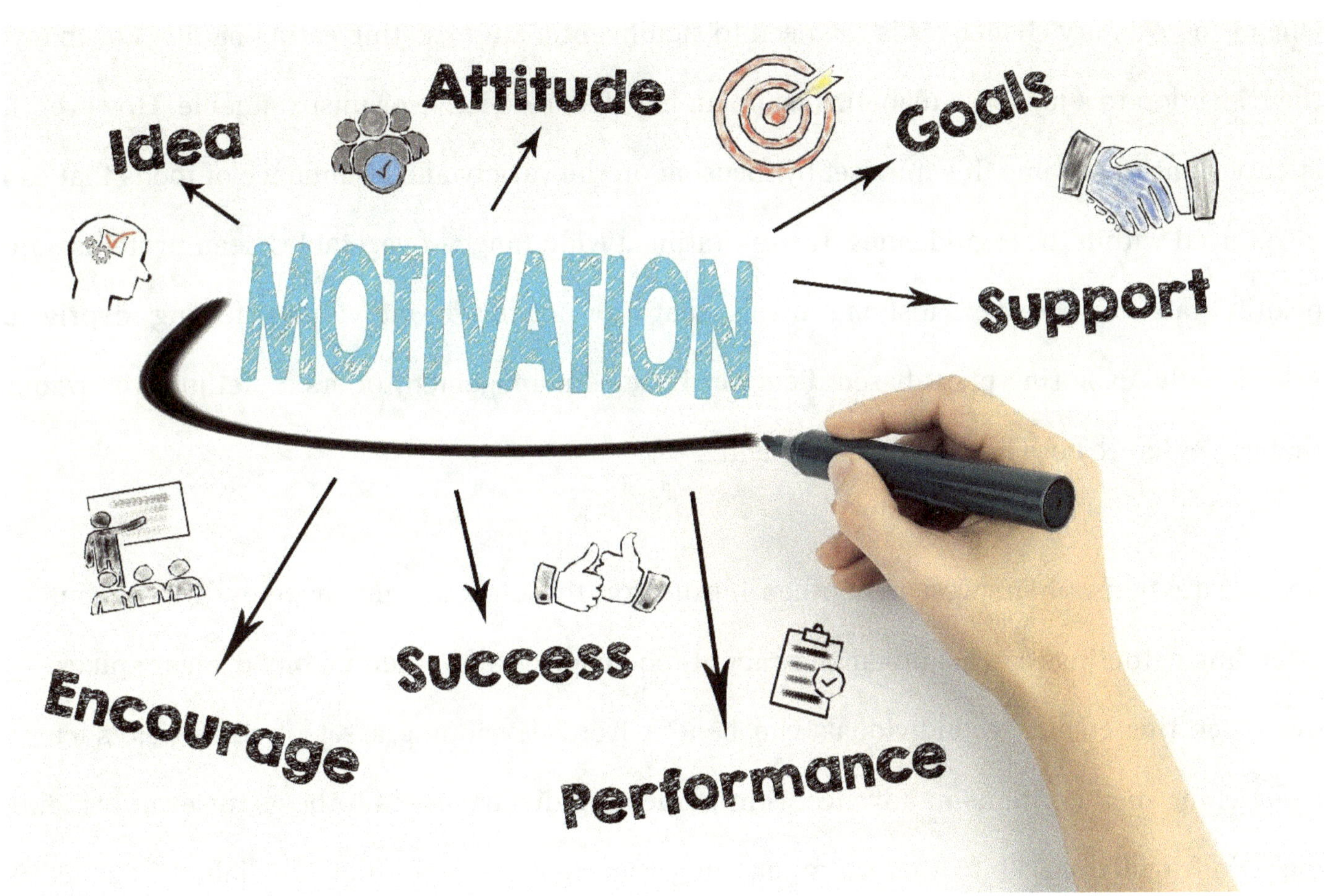

Overcoming Challenges

Overcoming challenges in managing diabetes requires a multifaceted approach that addresses dietary choices, lifestyle adjustments, and emotional resilience.

Individuals navigating a diabetic diet often face hurdles such as resistance to change, cravings for high-carb foods, and the overwhelming nature of meal planning. Acknowledging these challenges is the first step towards developing effective strategies that promote adherence to a diabetic-friendly lifestyle. Understanding the psychological and emotional aspects of dietary change is crucial, as it can significantly impact one's ability to stick to a meal plan.

One of the primary challenges is the need to significantly alter existing eating habits. For many, the transition to a low-carb diabetic meal plan may feel restrictive or unsustainable. However, it is important to reframe this mindset by focusing on the variety and abundance of foods that can be enjoyed within these guidelines. Incorporating a wide range of vegetables, lean proteins, and healthy fats can create satisfying meals that do not leave individuals feeling deprived. Additionally, exploring plant-based diets for diabetes management offers a plethora of options that can enhance both health and enjoyment.

Social situations often present another hurdle for those managing diabetes. Dining out or attending gatherings can lead to anxiety about food choices and potential blood sugar spikes. To overcome this challenge, individuals can benefit from developing a set of strategies, such as researching menu options in advance, communicating dietary needs to hosts, or even bringing diabetic-friendly snacks to share. Emphasizing the Mediterranean diet for diabetics, which is rich in vegetables, whole grains, and lean proteins, can also provide a balanced approach that aligns with social dining experiences without compromising health.

Meal preparation is a crucial element in maintaining a diabetic-friendly diet, yet it can be time-consuming and daunting for many. Establishing a consistent meal prep strategy can alleviate stress and promote healthier choices throughout the week.

By dedicating time to plan and prepare meals in advance, individuals can ensure they have access to nutritious options, reducing the temptation to resort to convenience foods that may not align with their dietary needs. Utilizing diabetic-friendly recipes, including gluten-free options, can enhance creativity in the kitchen while adhering to dietary restrictions.

Lastly, the emotional aspect of managing diabetes should not be overlooked. The journey can often feel isolating, and individuals may experience feelings of frustration or defeat. Engaging with supportive communities, whether online or in-person, can provide encouragement and motivation. Furthermore, exploring intermittent fasting as a tool for diabetes control can empower individuals to take charge of their health while navigating challenges. By embracing a proactive mindset and seeking out resources, individuals can successfully navigate the complexities of diabetes management and cultivate a fulfilling, healthy lifestyle.

Setting Realistic Goals

Setting realistic goals is a fundamental aspect of successfully managing diabetes through diet. For individuals embarking on a diabetic diet, whether they lean towards low-carb meal plans, plant-based diets, or the Mediterranean approach, it is essential to establish achievable targets that align with their lifestyle and health needs. This practice not only fosters motivation but also supports long-term adherence to dietary changes. When setting these goals, consideration should be given to individual circumstances, resources, and preferences to ensure they are both attainable and relevant.

A critical first step in goal setting is assessing current dietary habits and identifying areas for improvement. For instance, those accustomed to high-carb meals may find it challenging to switch immediately to a low-carb diet.

Instead, a more realistic approach would involve gradually reducing carbohydrate intake over several weeks. This could include replacing refined carbohydrates with whole grains or exploring diabetic-friendly snack options that satisfy cravings without compromising blood sugar levels. Such incremental changes can facilitate a smoother transition and instill a sense of accomplishment as each small goal is met.

In addition to focusing on food choices, it is vital to incorporate aspects of meal planning and preparation into the goal-setting process. Developing diabetic meal prep strategies can simplify daily cooking and help individuals maintain their dietary guidelines. Setting specific objectives, such as preparing meals in advance for the week or experimenting with gluten-free diabetic recipes, can lead to greater consistency in adhering to a diabetic diet. By making meal prep a priority, individuals can reduce the temptation to resort to unhealthy options when time is limited or when faced with cravings.

Intermittent fasting has gained popularity as a method for diabetes control and can be effectively integrated into realistic goal setting. Individuals interested in this approach should start by defining manageable fasting periods that suit their lifestyle. For example, beginning with a 12-hour fasting window and gradually extending it can help the body adapt without feeling overwhelmed. This method not only aids in blood sugar management but also encourages mindfulness regarding food choices during eating periods, making it easier to select diabetes-friendly desserts and low-carb meals.

Lastly, culturally specific diabetic diets can play a significant role in keeping individuals motivated and engaged with their dietary goals. Embracing traditional foods that align with diabetes management can enhance satisfaction and compliance. Setting goals around exploring new recipes that fit within one's cultural context, while ensuring they meet diabetic guidelines, can create a sense of connection and enjoyment in the diet.

It is essential to recognize that realistic goals are not solely about restriction; they should also celebrate the diverse culinary options available for those managing diabetes, promoting a balanced and fulfilling approach to eating.

Finding Support and Community

Finding a supportive community is essential for individuals managing diabetes, as it can significantly enhance both emotional well-being and dietary adherence. Whether you are a man or a woman, connecting with others who share similar experiences can provide encouragement, accountability, and valuable insights into living with diabetes. Support can come from various sources, including healthcare professionals, online forums, local support groups, or friends and family who understand the challenges and triumphs associated with managing a diabetic diet.

Online forums and social media groups have become popular platforms for individuals seeking support and information regarding diabetic diets. These virtual communities allow members to share personal experiences, recipes, and tips on low-carb diabetic meal plans or plant-based diets tailored for diabetes management. Engaging in discussions about Mediterranean diets or gluten-free recipes can lead to discovering new meal ideas, snacks, and dessert options that align with specific dietary needs. The ability to reach out to others facing similar challenges can foster a sense of belonging and reduce feelings of isolation.

Local diabetes support groups can also play a pivotal role in building community. These gatherings often feature guest speakers, cooking demonstrations, and discussions surrounding various diabetic diets and meal prep strategies. Attending these meetings can provide face-to-face interaction, allowing individuals to form lasting relationships and support networks.

Furthermore, sharing experiences in a safe environment can empower members to adopt healthier lifestyle changes, such as exploring intermittent fasting methods or incorporating nutritional supplements into their daily routine.

For those interested in culturally specific diabetic diets, joining community organizations or cultural groups can be particularly beneficial. These groups often provide resources and support tailored to specific cultural backgrounds, ensuring that dietary choices remain relevant and feasible. By participating in cooking classes or potlucks, individuals can learn how to adapt traditional recipes to be more diabetes-friendly, while also enjoying the comfort of familiar flavors. This not only strengthens cultural ties but also enhances the collective knowledge of managing diabetes within that community.

Ultimately, finding support and community in the journey of managing diabetes can significantly impact one's approach to diet and lifestyle. By leveraging both online and offline resources, individuals can cultivate a network of peers who understand the intricacies of diabetic nutrition. Whether navigating meal prep strategies or exploring the world of diabetes-friendly desserts, having a supportive community fosters resilience and encourages individuals to stay committed to their health goals.

Chapter 19: Resources for Continued Learning

Recommended Books and Websites

For individuals seeking to deepen their understanding of diabetic diets and meal planning, numerous books and websites serve as invaluable resources. These materials cater to a variety of needs, from foundational knowledge about diabetes management to specific dietary approaches such as low-carb, plant-based, and Mediterranean diets. A thorough exploration of these resources can empower readers to make informed choices that align with their health goals.

One highly recommended book is "The Complete Guide to Fasting" by Dr. Jason Fung. This book provides a comprehensive overview of intermittent fasting, which has been shown to aid in diabetes control. It discusses the science behind fasting and offers practical tips for integrating it into one's lifestyle. Readers can benefit from understanding the various fasting protocols and how they can be tailored to fit their individual needs, making it an essential addition to any diabetic's library.

For those interested in plant-based diets, "Plant-Based Diet for Dummies" by Marni Wasserman offers a wealth of information. This book outlines the benefits of a plant-based approach for diabetes management and provides delicious, diabetic-friendly recipes. It emphasizes the importance of whole foods and nutrient density, helping readers make healthier choices while enjoying satisfying meals. This resource is particularly useful for individuals looking to incorporate more fruits, vegetables, and legumes into their diets.

Websites such as the American Diabetes Association (ADA) offer a plethora of information related to diabetes-friendly eating. The ADA website features meal plans, recipes, and articles on various dietary strategies, including gluten-free options and culturally specific diets. Additionally, it provides access to research and guidelines that can aid individuals in navigating their dietary choices. The interactive nature of the website allows users to explore topics relevant to their personal dietary needs.

Lastly, " The Complete Diabetes Cookbook" by the America's Test Kitchen is an excellent resource for anyone looking to explore diabetic-friendly desserts, soups and snacks options. This cookbook includes a variety of recipes that are both satisfying and compliant with diabetic dietary guidelines. It focuses on portion control, balanced nutrition, and creative meal prep strategies, making it a practical guide for anyone looking to maintain a healthy lifestyle while managing diabetes. By utilizing these books and websites, readers can enhance their knowledge and skills in creating delicious, diabetes-friendly meals.

Meal Prep Apps and Tools

Meal prep apps and tools have become essential resources for individuals managing diabetes. These digital platforms not only streamline the meal planning process but also cater specifically to the dietary needs of diabetics. Users can easily input their preferences, such as low-carb or plant-based options, and the apps will generate customized meal plans that align with their health goals. This functionality is particularly beneficial for those adhering to specific diets, such as the Mediterranean diet, as the apps can provide recipes and shopping lists tailored to these nutritional frameworks.

Incorporating meal prep tools into diabetic meal management can significantly enhance adherence to dietary recommendations. Many apps offer features that allow users to track their carbohydrate intake, monitor their blood sugar levels, and even connect with healthcare providers for personalized advice. This integration of technology aids individuals in making informed food choices, ensuring that they remain within their dietary limits while still enjoying a variety of meals. Furthermore, the ability to plan meals in advance reduces the likelihood of impulsive eating decisions, a common challenge for those managing diabetes.

Meal prep apps also facilitate the exploration of diabetic-friendly snack options and desserts. Users can access a wealth of recipes that cater to their specific dietary restrictions, including gluten-free and low-carb variations. This variety is crucial for maintaining interest in meal planning and preventing dietary fatigue. By utilizing these tools, individuals can discover new favorites and incorporate culturally specific dishes into their repertoire, making healthy eating both enjoyable and sustainable.

Another advantage of using meal prep apps is their ability to assist with intermittent fasting strategies. Many of these platforms provide guidance on how to structure meals and snacks within designated eating windows. This can be particularly helpful for those looking to maintain stable blood sugar levels while following fasting protocols. The apps can suggest recipes that are not only diabetes-friendly but also filling and satisfying, ensuring that users feel nourished during their eating periods.

Lastly, in the realm of nutritional supplements, meal prep apps often include features that allow users to track their supplement intake alongside their meals. This holistic approach helps individuals ensure they are meeting their nutritional needs while managing diabetes.

By combining meal planning with supplement tracking, these tools empower users to take control of their health journey, making it easier to adhere to their dietary goals and improve overall well-being. Integrating technology into meal preparation fosters a proactive approach to diabetes management, ultimately leading to better health outcomes.

Joining Diabetes Support Groups

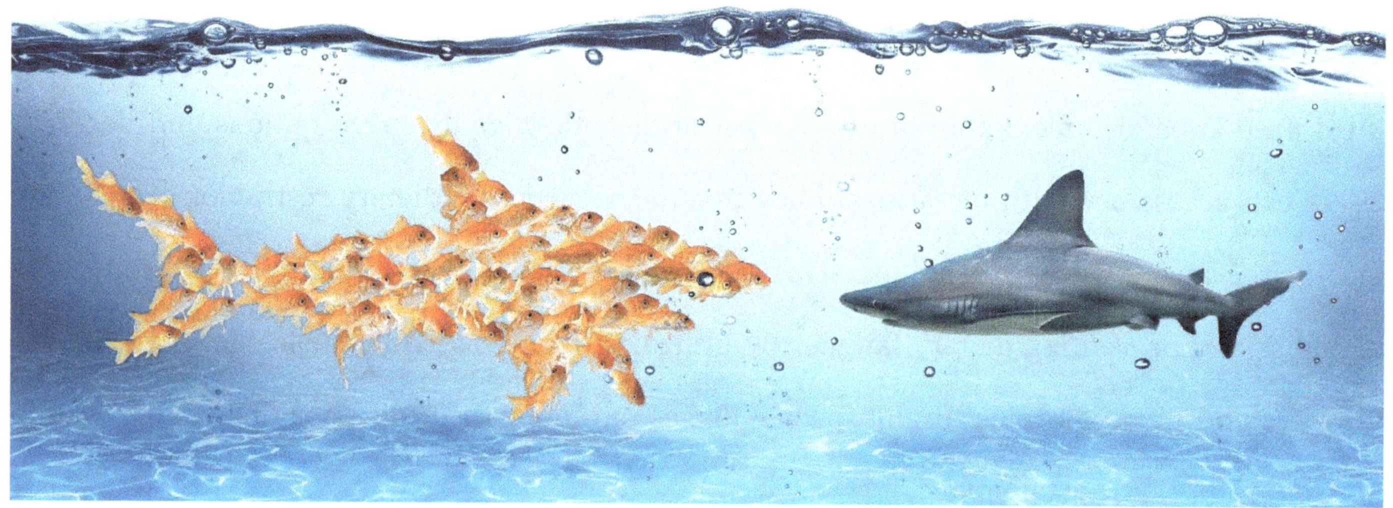

Joining a diabetes support group can significantly enhance the journey of individuals managing diabetes. These groups provide a platform for sharing experiences, exchanging tips, and discovering effective strategies for maintaining a diabetic diet. For both men and women, the emotional and practical aspects of living with diabetes can be overwhelming, and support groups often serve as a lifeline. They foster a sense of community, allowing participants to connect with others who understand the daily challenges and triumphs associated with diabetes management. Support groups often focus on specific dietary approaches that may resonate with different members. For instance, those interested in low-carb meal plans can engage in discussions around meal preparation strategies that are both enjoyable and compliant with their dietary needs.

The exchange of diabetic-friendly recipes, including gluten-free and plant-based options, allows members to explore diverse culinary avenues that can contribute to better health outcomes. Sharing insights on Mediterranean diets or culturally specific dietary practices can also enrich the group's collective knowledge and foster inclusivity.

Moreover, support groups can be instrumental in addressing psychological aspects of diabetes management. The emotional support offered by peers can alleviate feelings of isolation and stress, which are common among those living with chronic conditions. Engaging in conversations about intermittent fasting for diabetes control or nutritional supplements can empower individuals to take charge of their health. These discussions often lead to increased motivation and adherence to dietary recommendations, as members encourage one another to explore new approaches to meal planning and health management.

Participation in a support group also provides access to expert guidance. Many groups invite healthcare professionals to share their expertise on various topics, including managing blood sugar levels, meal prep strategies, and the benefits of specific diets.

This access to credible information can help demystify the complexities of diabetes management and reinforce the importance of adhering to personalized dietary plans. It can also create opportunities for members to ask questions and gain insights tailored to their unique health situations.

In conclusion, joining a diabetes support group can be a transformative experience for individuals navigating the complexities of diabetes management. The shared experiences, diverse dietary strategies, and emotional support available within these groups can empower members to take proactive steps toward achieving their health goals. Whether exploring diabetic-friendly desserts or discussing the latest research on nutrition, the connections formed in these groups can enrich each member's journey, making the path to diabetes management more manageable and enjoyable.

Conclusion

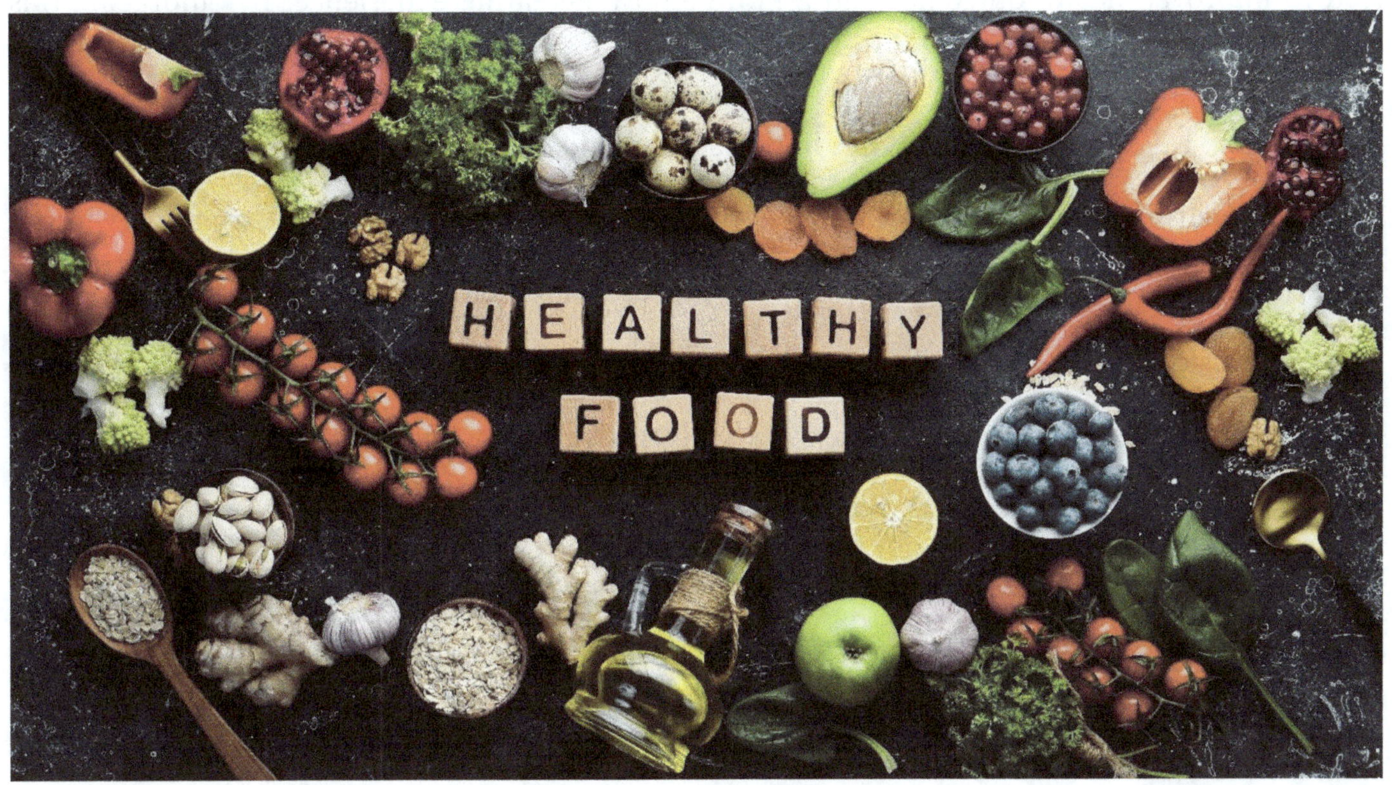

In conclusion, embarking on a diabetic diet journey requires a multifaceted approach that not only addresses the nutritional needs but also considers personal preferences and lifestyle choices. This cookbook has aimed to provide you with diverse recipes and meal plans that cater to various niches within the diabetic community. From low-carb options to plant-based meals, we have emphasized the importance of balancing carbohydrate intake while ensuring that each meal remains enjoyable and satisfying. Understanding the significance of food as both nourishment and pleasure is essential for maintaining a healthy lifestyle while managing diabetes effectively.

The Mediterranean diet stands out as a sustainable and heart-healthy option for individuals with diabetes. Its emphasis on whole foods, healthy fats, and lean proteins provides a rich variety of flavors and textures.

We encourage you to explore these recipes, as they not only support blood sugar management but also promote overall well-being. Incorporating elements of the Mediterranean lifestyle can lead to improved health outcomes and a more enjoyable eating experience. By embracing this diet, you are not just managing diabetes; you are also enhancing your quality of life.

In addition, we have highlighted the importance of diabetic-friendly snacks and gluten-free options, ensuring that you have a range of choices that fit your dietary restrictions without compromising taste. Snack time can be a challenging moment for many, but with the right recipes and strategies, you can enjoy satisfying treats that align with your health goals. Whether it's a quick nibble or a planned snack, the recipes provided encourage mindful eating and can help stabilize blood sugar levels throughout the day.

Meal prep strategies play a crucial role in maintaining a diabetic diet. By preparing meals in advance, you gain control over your food choices and reduce the temptation to opt for less healthy options. This cookbook offers practical tips and recipes that simplify the meal preparation process, making it easier to adhere to your dietary plan. Dedicating time to meal prep not only saves you effort during busy weekdays but also fosters a sense of accomplishment and commitment to your health journey.

Lastly, we encourage you to explore culturally specific diabetic diets and consider the nutritional supplements that could enhance your dietary approach. Each culture offers unique ingredients and preparation methods that can contribute to a balanced diabetic meal plan. Adapting these elements into your diet can make your journey more personalized and enjoyable. As you move forward, remember that diabetes management is a continuous process, and with the knowledge and tools provided in this cookbook, you are well-equipped to create a delicious, fulfilling, and health-conscious culinary experience.

SCAN THE QR CODE